Progress in Pathology

Volume 5

Edited by

Nigel Kirkham MD FRCPath
Consultant Histopathologist
Royal Sussex County Hospital
Brighton

Nicholas R Lemoine PhD MD MRCPath
ICRF Molecular Oncology Unit
Hammersmith Hospital
London

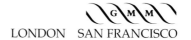
LONDON   SAN FRANCISCO

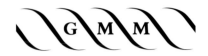

Greenwich Medical Media Limited
137 Euston Road
London
NW1 2AA

870 Market Street, Ste 720
San Francisco
CA 94109

ISBN 1 8411 00 501

First published 2001

Distributed worldwide by Plymbridge Distributors Ltd
and in the USA by Jamco Distribution

Typeset by Saxon Graphics Ltd, Derby
Printed in China

Visit our website at:
www.greenwich-medical.co.uk

Contents

Contributors

Tracey A. Bailey BSc (Hons), PhD
Post-doctoral Scientist
Department of Pathology
Institute of Ophthalmology
University College London
UK

Leigh R . Biddlestone PhD
Consultant Histopathologist and
    Cytopathologist
Southmead Hospital
Westbury-on-Trym
Bristol,
UK

J. J. Boyle BSc, MB ChB
MRC Training Fellow
Departments of Histopathology and
    Medicine
Addenbrooke's Hospital
Cambridge,
UK

Lorenzo Cerroni MD
Associate Professor of Dermatology
Department of Dermatology
University of Graz
Austria

Alistair J. Cochran MD FRCPath,
    FRCP(Glas)
Professor of Pathology and Surgery
Department of Pathology and Laboratory
    Medicine
UCLA School of Medicine
Los Angeles, California
USA

M. Giles S. Dunnill MD, MRCP
Consultant Dermatologist
Bristol Royal Infirmary
Bristol,
UK

Patrick J. Gallagher
Reader / Consultant Histopathologist
Southampton University Hospitals
Southampton,
UK

Deirdre Mary Guerin MB, BCh, BAO,
    MRCPath, DipRCPath (Derm)
Consultant Dermatopathologist
Department of Histopathology
Royal Liverpool University Hospital
Liverpool,
UK

Yuji Itai MD, PhD
Professor
Institute of Clinical Medicine
University of Tsukuba
Ibaraki,
Japan

Helmut Kerl MD
Professor and Chairman
Department of Dermatology
University of Graz
Austria

Nigel Kirkham MD FRCPath
Consultant Histopathologist
Royal Sussex County Hospital
Brighton,
UK

Irene M. Leigh MD, FRCP
Professor of Dermatology
Centre for Cutaneous Research
St Bartholomew's and the Royal London
    School of Medicine and Dentistry
Queen Mary and Westfield College
Clinical Sciences and Research Centre
London,
UK

George B. M. Lindop BSc, MB, ChB,
    FRCP (Glasg), FRCPath
Reader in Pathology
University of Glasgow Department of
    Pathology
Western Infirmary
Glasgow,
UK

James A. Morris MA, MB, BChir,
    FRCPath
Consultant Pathologist
Department of Pathology
Royal Lancaster Infirmary
Lancaster,
UK

Neil A. Shepherd MBBS, FRCPath
Consultant Histopathologist
Department of Histopathology
Gloucester Royal Hospital
Gloucester,
UK

Tohoru Takeda MD
Assistant Professor
Institute of Clinical Medicine
University of Tsukuba
Ibaraki,
Japan

Suzanne Wakely
Senior House Officer
Department of Medicine
Royal Bournemouth Hospital
Bournemouth,
UK

Janine Wechsler MD
Department of Pathology
Henri Mondor Hospital
Creteil,
France

Cheryl E. Whittles Former PhD student
Biotechnology Centre and
    The Gloucestershire Royal Hospital
    and Cranfield Institute of
    Medical Sciences
Cranfield University,
UK

Judy Wyatt MB ChB, FRCPath
Consultant Histopathologist
St James's University Hospital
Leeds,
UK

Preface

Volume 5 of *Progress in Pathology* sees us with a new publisher, but the formula remains the same. We aim to bring you a collection of interesting, thought provoking and useful chapters. In this volume we have three chapters on difficult areas in dermatopathology as well as a timely review on the sentinel node biopsy: a procedure that is likely to become very widely used in the near future, especially if its value is supported by the clinical trials currently under way.

Other contributions cover aspects Barratt's oesophagus and the routine reporting of non-neoplastic gastric biopsies. The potentially useful technique of X-ray micro-computed tomography is described. The molecular basis of inherited skin disorders is reviewed and put into its clinical context. The importance of arterial remodelling is reviewed. The volume concludes with discussions of how errors may occur in histopathology and of aspects of the mathematical basis of diagnosis.

We feel confident that this volume will make a good read and a useful reference. We look forward to bringing the next volume to you when we will all be established in the third millenium.

Brighton N.K.
London N.R.L.
2001

1

The clinicopathological spectrum of cutaneous B-cell lymphomas

Lorenzo Cerroni   Helmut Kerl

In the past, studies on malignant lymphoproliferative disorders of the skin were concerned mainly with lymphomas of the T-cell type. In recent years, through the synthesis of classical morphological studies and progress in immunology and molecular biology, it has been recognized that B-cell lymphomas that arise in the skin (primary cutaneous B-cell lymphomas or PCBCLs) represent a distinct and very important group of extranodal lymphomas.[1] They occur far more frequently than was generally believed. The widespread use of immunohistochemical and molecular genetic techniques has revealed that many of the cases classified in the past as cutaneous B-cell pseudolymphomas in fact represent low-grade malignant B-cell lymphomas of the skin.[2,3]

It is extremely important to emphasize that the treatment strategies for PCBCLs are completely different from those applied to other malignant lymphomas. It is therefore crucial to distinguish PCBCLs from secondary cutaneous manifestations of extracutaneous (usually nodal) B-cell lymphomas. PCBCL is defined as the presence of cutaneous disease alone with no evidence of extracutaneous spread over a period of at least 6 months after complete staging procedures.[4,5]

There are still many problems relating to the classification of PCBCLs. Some authors maintain that they represent, for the most part, B-cell lymphomas of germinal centre cell origin, whereas others believe that the majority consist of marginal zone, lymphomas of mucosa-associated lymphoid tissue-like (MALT-like) lymphomas.[6-9] There is also a view that all PCBCLs should be classified as skin-associated lymphoid tissue-type ('SALT-type B-cell lymphoma'), irrespective of morphological immunophenotypical and molecular patterns.[10] A classification of PCBCLs has been recently proposed by the Cutaneous Lymphoma Study Group of the European Organization for Research and Treatment of Cancer (EORTC) (Table 1.1).[4]

Lorenzo Cerroni MD, Associate Professor of Dermatology, Department of Dermatology, University of Graz, Auenbruggerplatz, 8, A-8036 Graz, Austria

Helmut Kerl MD, Professor and Chairman, Department of Dermatology, University of Graz, Avuenbruggerplatz, 8, A-8036 Graz, Austria

Table 1.1 EORTC classification of cutaneous lymphomas[4]

T-cell lymphomas	B-cell lymphomas
Indolent behaviour	*Indolent behaviour*
Mycosis fungoides	Follicle centre cell lymphoma
Mycosis fungoides with follicular mucinosis	Immunocytoma (marginal zone B-cell lymphoma)
Pagetoid reticulosis	
Large cell cutaneous T-cell lymphoma, CD30+	
Anaplastic	
Immunoblastic	
Pleomorphic	
Lymphomatoid papulosis	
Aggressive behaviour	*Intermediate behaviour*
Sézary syndrome	Large B-cell lymphoma of the leg
Large cell T-cell lymphomas, CD30-	
Immunoblastic	
Pleomorphic	
*Provisional entities**	*Provisional entities**
Granulomatous slack skin	Intravascular large B-cell lymphoma
CTCL, pleomorphic small/medium-sized	Plasmacytoma
Subcutaneous panniculitis-like T-cell lymphoma	

*This group includes cutaneous lymphomas with insufficient data to delineate clear-cut clinicopathological entities.
CTCL = Cutaneous T-cell Lymphoma

Table 1.2 Antibodies useful for the diagnosis of cutaneous lymphoproliferative diseases in routinely-fixed, paraffin-embedded tissue sections

Antibody	CD	Source	Main specificity
PS1	3	Novocastra	Pan-T lymphocytes
I290	4	Novocastra	T-helper lymphocytes
54/B4	5	Novocastra	T lymphocytes, B-CLL
C8/144b	8	Dako	T-suppressor lymphocytes
270	10	Novocastra	CALLA, germinal centre cells
C3D-1	15	Dako	Reed-Sternberg cells, myeloid cells
L26	20	Dako	B lymphocytes
1F8	21	Dako	Dendritic reticulum cells
BerH2	30	Dako	Activated lymphocytes, Reed-Sternberg cells
DF-T1	43	Dako	T lymphocytes, monocytes, myeloid cells
UCHL1	45RO	Dako	T lymphocytes, monocytes, myeloid cells
N-CAM16	56	Novocastra	NK cells
PGM1	68	Dako	Monocytes/macrophages, myeloid cells
mb-1	79a	Dako	B-lymphocytes, plasmacells
mic-2	99	Dako	Leucocytes, Ewing's sarcoma
Ig		Dako	Immunoglobulin heavy and light chains
S100		Dako	T-zone histiocytes
MIB1		Dianova	Proliferating cells
124		Dako	*bcl-2* protein
TdT		Dako	Precursor lymphocytes
TIA-1		Coulter	Cytotoxic lymphocytes
Granzyme-B		Monosan	Cytotoxic lymphocytes
ALK-1		Dako	t(2;5) fusion protein
CS1-4		Dako	EBV-latent membrane protein

All antibodies are to be used after antigen retrieval treatment (heat retrieval).
B-CLL = B-cell chronic lymphocytic leukaemia; CALLA = common acute lymphoblastic leukemia antigen; NK = natural killer; EBV = Esptein-Barr virus.

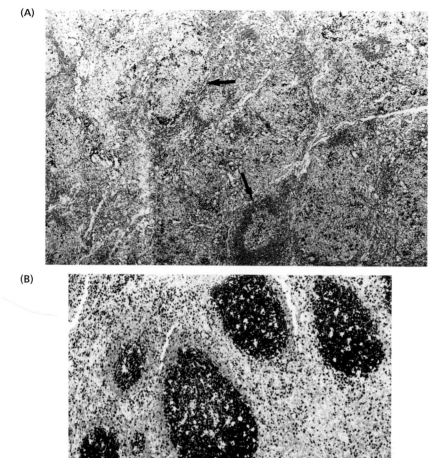

Fig. 1.2 (A) Cutaneous follicle centre lymphoma, follicular; note low proliferation rate within neoplastic follicles as detected by immunohistology (arrows) (antibody MIB-1). **(B)** By contrast, reactive germinal centres within a tonsil display a strong MIB-1 positivity.

Clinically patients present with recurrent red to reddish-brown papules, plaques and nodules localized preferentially on the upper extremities or the trunk. Generalized lesions can be observed in a minority of patients. The prognosis is excellent. In a recent study no patient showed internal involvement after a mean follow-up of more than 4 years.[3]

HISTOPATHOLOGY

Histology shows patchy, nodular or diffuse infiltrates involving the dermis and subcutaneous fat.[3] The epidermis is spared. A characteristic pattern can be observed at low power: nodular infiltrates, sometimes containing reactive germinal centres, are surrounded by a pale-staining population of small to medium-sized cells with indented nuclei, inconspicuous nucleoli and abundant pale cytoplasm (variously described as marginal zone cells, centrocyte-like cells, or monocytoid B-cells) (Fig. 1.3). In addition, plasma cells (at the margins of the infiltrate), lymphoplasmacytoid cells, small lymphocytes and occasional large blasts are observed. Eosinophils are also a common finding. In some cases there may be a granulomatous reaction with epitheloid- and giant cells.

The centrocyte-like cells reveal positivity for CD20, CD79a and Bcl-2, and negativity for CD5 and CD10. In about 65% of cases, intracytoplasmic monotypical expression of immunoglobulin light chains can be observed. The monoclonal population of B lymphocytes is characteristically arranged at the periphery of cellular aggregates (Fig. 1.4). Staining with the monocytoid B-cell-related antibody Ki-M1p shows a positive reactivity of neoplastic cells with a characteristic intra-

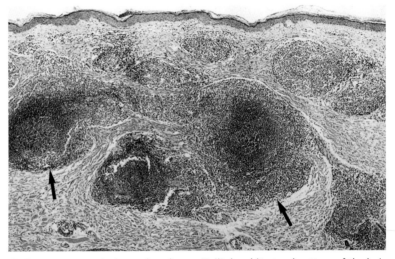

Fig. 1.3 Cutaneous marginal zone lymphoma. Typical architectural pattern of the lesion characterized by nodular infiltrates, sometimes containing reactive germinal centres, surrounded by a pale staining population of small to medium-sized cells with indented nuclei, inconspicuous nucleoli and abundant pale cytoplasm (arrows).

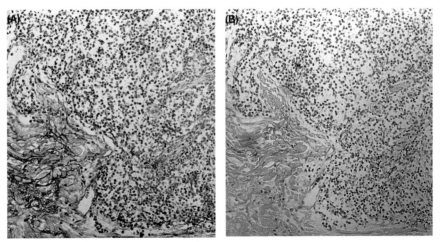

Fig. 1.4 Cutaneous marginal zone lymphoma. **(A)** monoclonal expression of immunoglobulin light chain kappa. **(B)** immunohistochemical reaction for immunoglobulin light chain lambda is negative.

cytoplasmic granular pattern. Monoclonal rearrangement of the J_H genes can be observed in the majority of cases.

CUTANEOUS IMMUNOCYTOMA

Cutaneous immunocytoma is defined as a proliferation of small lymphocytes, lymphoplasmacytoid cells and plasma cells with monotypical intracytoplasmic immunoglobulins. Primary cutaneous immunocytoma differs from nodal immunocytoma in that patients do not show features of Waldenström's macroglobulinæmia, and have an excellent prognosis and response to treatment.[27] Some authors consider immunocytoma and MZL of the skin to be a single entity of low-grade malignant cutaneous B-cell lymphoma.[10,28]

Clinically patients present with solitary, or grouped, erythematous to reddish-brown plaques or dome-shaped tumours that are found especially on the lower extremities. Generalized lesions are rare. Immunocytoma can arise in skin areas affected by acrodermatitis chronica atrophicans, and may be linked to infection by *B. burgdorferi*. In fact, *B. burgdorferi* DNA sequences have been demonstrated using PCR analysis in cutaneous lesions from three out of four patients tested.[12] The prognosis is excellent, although local recurrences can be observed.

HISTOPATHOLOGY

The architectural pattern is characterized by dense, monomorphous, nodular or diffuse infiltrates with involvement of the dermis and subcutis (Fig. 1.5).[3,29] The

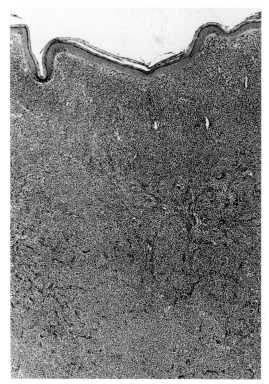

Fig. 1.5 Cutaneous immunocytoma. Dense, homogeneous proliferation of small to medium-sized cells.

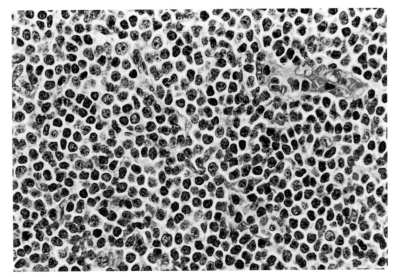

Fig. 1.6 Cutaneous immunocytoma. Lymphoplasmacytoid cells admixed with small lymphocytes and a few blasts.

epidermis is usually spared. The predominating cell types are lymphoplasmacytoid cells and small lymphocytes (Fig. 1.6). In addition, plasma cells are usually present, often located at the periphery of the infiltrates. Periodic acid Schiff-positive intranuclear inclusions (Dutcher bodies) are observed sometimes and represent a valuable diagnostic clue. Reactive germinal centres can be found in a few cases.

Neoplastic cells express monoclonal cytoplasmic immunoglobulins in most cases. In contrast to nodal immunocytoma, which is characterized by intracytoplasmic IgM, cutaneous lesions more often show IgG positivity. Cells are positive for CD20, CD79a and Bcl-2, and negative for CD5. An aberrant positivity for CD43 is found in about 50% of cases. Molecular analysis reveals monoclonal rearrangement of the J_H gene in most lesions.

CUTANEOUS PLASMACYTOMA

Cutaneous plasmacytoma is a B-cell lymphoma that is characterized by the clonal proliferation of plasma cells primarily affecting the skin, in the absence of bone marrow involvement (extramedullary plasmacytoma).[30,31] This type of cutaneous B-cell lymphoma is exceedingly rare.

Patients present clinically with solitary, clustered, or, in exceptional cases, generalized erythematous, reddish-brown or violaceous cutaneous/subcutaneous plaques or tumours. There is a predilection for the head and trunk. Cutaneous plasmacytoma occurs mostly in elderly male patients. The prognosis is controversial. In fact, although some reports have claimed that solitary lesions have a very good prognosis, comparable to that of solitary extramedullary plasmacytoma arising in other tissues, the development of multiple myeloma or systemic soft-tissue metastases have been observed in some patients.

HISTOPATHOLOGY

The tumour consists of dense nodules and/or sheets of cells within the entire dermis and subcutis (Fig. 1.7).[32] Mature and immature plasma cells with varying degrees of atypia predominate (Fig. 1.8). Dutcher bodies and Russell bodies are found occasionally. Small, reactive lymphocytes are few or absent. In a few cases

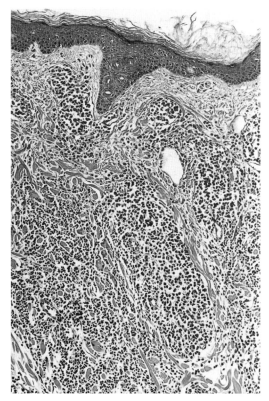

Fig. 1.7 Cutaneous plasmacytoma. Nodules of plasma cells within the dermis.

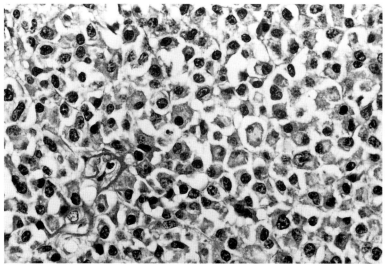

Fig. 1.8 Cutaneous plasmacytoma. Typical and atypical plasma cells predominate.

amyloid deposits are present within and/or surrounding the neoplastic infiltrates. Crystalloid intracytoplasmic inclusions within histiocytes and macrophages may also occur.

Neoplastic plasma cells contain cIg (usually IgA) and show monoclonal expression of one immunoglobulin light chain. CD45 and most B-cell-associated markers are negative, but cells are positive for CD38 in most cases and, less frequently, for CD79a. Immunohistochemical expression of cytokeratins, HMB45 and CD30, can be observed within neoplastic plasma cells, representing the source of a pitfall in diagnosis. Molecular analysis usually reveals a monoclonal rearrangement of the J_H gene.

Primary cutaneous plasmacytoma must be differentiated from reactive plasma cell proliferations and from cutaneous inflammatory pseudotumour (plasma cell granuloma).[33] In reactive conditions plasma cells are not atypical, and display a polyclonal pattern of immunoglobulin light chain expression.

LARGE B-CELL LYMPHOMA OF THE LEG

Large B-cell lymphoma of the leg (LBCL) represents a primary cutaneous B-cell lymphoma that is characterized by large cell morphology and intermediate prognosis, and that occurs almost exclusively in elderly patients, predominantly females. The prognosis is more unfavourable than in other types of PCBCL, with a 5-year survival rate of approximately 50% .[34]

Clinically patients present with solitary or clustered erythematous or reddish-brown nodules, mostly located on the distal extremity of one leg. Ulceration is common. Small erythematous papules can be seen adjacent to larger nodules. Tumours with similar morphological features can also arise on body areas other than the lower extremities.

HISTOPATHOLOGY

There is a dense, diffuse infiltrate within the dermis and subcutis.[34] The infiltrate involves usually the entire papillary dermis. Involvement of the epidermis by large neoplastic cells, simulating a T-cell lymphoma, can be observed in rare cases (B-cell epidermotropism) (Fig. 1.9). The neoplastic infiltrate consists predominantly of immunoblasts and centroblasts. Reactive small lymphocytes are few or absent. Mitoses are frequent. It has been proposed that most cases of LBCL represent large cell lymphomas originating from lymphocytes of the germinal centre.

Neoplastic cells express monoclonal sIg and/or cIg. They are positive for B-cell markers and usually for Bcl-2, but there can be (partial) loss of antigen expression. The tumours reveal monoclonal rearrangement of the J_H genes. The t(14;18) is not present.

LBCL must be differentiated from anaplastic large cell lymphoma and from non-lymphoid tumours such as metastases among others. The clinicopathological pattern together with phenotypical and molecular features allow the correct classification of these lesions in most cases.

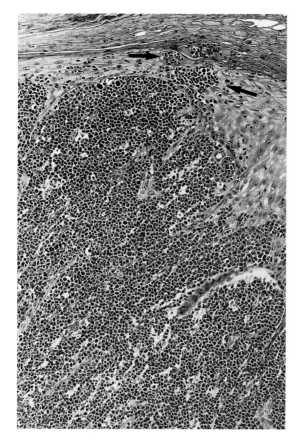

Fig. 1.9 Large B-cell lymphoma of the leg. Sheets of large B-lymphocytes predominate. Note intraepidermal collections of neoplastic cells simulating a cutaneous T-cell lymphoma (arrows).

INTRAVASCULAR LARGE B-CELL LYMPHOMA OF THE SKIN

Intravascular large B-cell lymphoma is a malignant proliferation of large B-lymphocytes within blood vessels.[35,36] This disease was formerly classified as a vascular neoplasm (malignant angioendotheliomatosis). Most cases show a B-cell phenotype, but a T-cell variant has been reported.[37] In rare patients the skin may be the only affected site, although more often there is systemic dissemination with common involvement of the central nervous system. It has been reported that the prognosis for intravascular large B-cell lymphoma that is limited to the skin is better than that for the generalized disease, but only a very limited number of cases have been observed.

Clinically patients present with indurated, erythematous or violaceous patches and plaques, preferentially located on the trunk and thighs. The clinical appearance is not typical of lymphoma, and may sometimes suggest a diagnosis of panniculitis or of purpura.

HISTOPATHOLOGY

Intravascular large B-cell lymphoma is characterized by a proliferation of large lymphocytes filling dilated blood vessels within the dermis and subcutaneous tissues.[38] In some cases atypical cells may also be observed around the blood vessels. The malignant cells are large with scanty cytoplasm and often prominent nucleoli. They are positive for B-cell-associated markers and express monoclonal sIg. Staining with endothelial cell-related antibodies (i.e. factor VIII, CD31, CD34) highlights the characteristic intravascular location of the cells. Molecular analysis shows monoclonal rearrangement of the J_H genes.

B-LYMPHOBLASTIC LYMPHOMA

B-lymphoblastic lymphomas are malignant proliferations of precursor B lymphocytes. Cases arising in the skin as the primary site have been observed only rarely.[39] It must be stressed that histological features alone do not allow the differentiation of lymphoblastic lymphomas with a B-cell phenotype from those of T-cell lineage.

Children and young adults are usually affected. Clinically patients present with large reddish tumours, commonly located on the head and neck.

HISTOPATHOLOGY

B-lymphoblastic lymphoma shows a monomorphous proliferation of medium-sized cells with scanty cytoplasm and round or convoluted nuclei with fine chromatin.[39] A 'starry sky' pattern is commonly seen at low power, due to the presence of macrophages with inclusion bodies ('tingible bodies'). Mitoses and necrotic cells are abundant. Immunohistology reveals reactivity for TdT, CD10, the cytoplasmic μ chain of immunoglobulins and, in most cases, for CD20 and CD79a. CD20 is negative in the pre-pre-B cell variant, which is positive for CD34. A proportion of cases also express CD43 and CD99. Molecular genetics usually shows a monoclonal rearrangement of the J_H genes and a polyclonal pattern for the T-cell receptor (TCR) genes, but polyclonality of J_H genes or monoclonal rearrangement of both TCR and J_H genes may be observed.

B-CELL CHRONIC LYMPHOCYTIC LEUKAEMIA

B-cell chronic lymphocytic leukaemia (B-CLL) represents the most common type of chronic lymphocytic leukaemia. Specific skin involvement is not rare, and in the past has sometimes been misinterpreted as 'cutaneous B-cell pseudolymphoma'.

Clinically patients present with localized or generalized erythematous papules, plaques or tumours. Peculiar clinical presentations include specific skin manifestations at sites of previous herpes simplex or herpes zoster eruptions, and massive involvement of the face producing the picture of the so-called 'facies leontina'.[40] Prognosis seems not to be affected by specific skin involvement.[41]

HISTOPATHOLOGY

Histology may show either a patchy perivascular and periadnexal pattern, or the presence of dense diffuse/nodular infiltrates of lymphocytes (Fig. 1.10).[41] As a

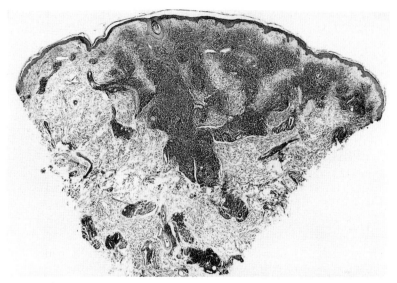

Fig. 1.10 Specific cutaneous infiltrate of B-cell chronic lymphocytic leukaemia. Dense infiltrate of neoplastic lymphocytes around vessels and adnexal structures involving the entire dermis and extending into the subcutaneous fat tissue.

rule, the subcutaneous fat tissue is involved. Cytomorphology reveals small lymphocytes without atypical features. Small nodular areas with larger cells showing features of prolymphocytes or paraimmunoblasts (so-called 'proliferation centres') can be observed occasionally. In many cases malignant B cells are admixed with other cell types such as T lymphocytes, eosinophils and epithelioid histiocytes.

Immunohistology reveals the presence of B lymphocytes characterized by an aberrant immunophenotype (CD20+, CD5+, CD43+) and monoclonal expression of immunoglobulin light chains. Molecular analysis shows, in most cases, a monoclonal rearrangement of the J_H genes.

RICHTER'S SYNDROME

Large cell transformation of B-CLL (Richter's syndrome) has been reported rarely in the skin. Patients present clinically with solitary, large cutaneous or subcutaneous tumours. Histology reveals features of a large B-cell lymphoma with predominance of centroblasts and immunoblasts. Immunohistology shows positivity for B-cell markers and monoclonal expression of immunoglobulin light chains. Molecular genetics confirms the presence of a monoclonal population of B lymphocytes. The clone may or may not be the same as that observed in the lymphocytes of the B-CLL, that is, at least in some cases, Richter's syndrome represents the occurrence of a high-grade lymphoma that is unrelated to the previous B-CLL (a so-called 'second lymphoma'). The prognosis for patients with cutaneous Richter's syndrome is very poor, and treatment is usually ineffective.

CONCLUSIONS

Very substantial guidelines and criteria for identifying PCBCLs are now available.[4,42,43] This has led to the reclassification of several cases that in the past were diagnosed as B-cell pseudolymphomas, and to the identification of various entities with well-defined clinicopathological features. Precise recognition of these entities will improve the diagnosis and therapy of cutaneous lymphomas.

KEY POINTS

- Primary cutaneous B-cell lymphomas are more frequent than previously recognized.
- Many cases diagnosed in the past as cutaneous B-cell pseudolymphoma are now classified among the cutaneous B-cell lymphomas of low-grade malignancy.
- It is crucial to distinguish primary cutaneous B-cell lymphomas from secondary cutaneous manifestations of extracutaneous (usually nodal) B-cell lymphomas, because prognostic features and treatment strategies are completely different.
- There are three main entities of low-grade malignancy primary cutaneous B-cell lymphoma (follicle centre lymphoma, marginal zone lymphoma and immunocytoma), which by some authors are reputed to belong to a single group of 'SALT-type' cutaneous B-cell lymphoma.
- The most important criteria for the differentiation of benign (reactive) from malignant skin infiltrates of B-lymphocytes are clinicopathological correlation and the detection of monoclonality by immunohistology, molecular biology, or both.
- It must be remembered that about one-third of cutaneous B-cell lymphoma cases neither reveals a monoclonal expression of immunoglobulin light chains by immunohistology, nor shows a monoclonal band by PCR analysis of the rearrangement of J_H genes.

REFERENCES

1. Kerl H, Kresbach H. Lymphoretikuläre Hyperplasien und Neoplasien der Haut. In: Schnyder UW (Ed.) Spezielle Pathologische Anatomie. Berlin, Springer Verlag, 1979; 396–399
2. Kerl H, Ackerman AB. Inflammatory diseases that simulate lymphomas: cutaneous pseudolymphomas. In: Fitzpatrick TB, Eisen AZ, Wolff K, Freedberg IM, Austen KF (Eds) Dermatology in General Medicine. 4th edn. New York: McGraw-Hill, Inc., 1993; 1315–1327
3. Cerroni L, Signoretti S, Höfler G et al. Primary cutaneous marginal zone B-cell lymphoma. A recently described entity of low-grade malignant cutaneous B-cell lymphoma. Am J Surg Pathol 1997; 21: 1307–1315
4. Willemze R, Kerl H, Sterry W et al. EORTC classification for primary cutaneous lymphomas: a proposal from the Cutaneous Lymphoma Study Group of the European Organization for Research and Treatment of Cancer. Blood 1997; 90: 354–371
5. Kerl H, Cerroni L. Primary B-cell lymphomas of the skin. Ann Oncol 1997; 8 (suppl. 2): 29–32

6. Willemze R, Rijlaarsdam JU, Beljaards RC, Meijer CJLM. Classification of primary cutaneous lymphomas. Historical overview and perspectives. Dermatology 1994; 189: 8–15

7. Pimpinelli N, Santucci M, Bosi A et al. Primary cutaneous follicular centre-cell lymphoma: a lymphoproliferative disease with favourable prognosis. Clin Exp Dermatol 1989; 14: 12–19

8. Slater DN. MALT and SALT: the clue to cutaneous B-cell lymphoproliferative disease. Br J Dermatol 1994; 131: 557–561

9. Isaacson PG, Norton AJ. Extranodal lymphomas. Edinburgh: Churchill Livingstone, 1994; see Cutaneous lymphoma pp. 172–176

10. Santucci M, Pimpinelli N, Arganini L. Primary cutaneous B-cell lymphoma: a unique type of low-grade lymphoma – clinicopathologic and immunologic study of 83 cases. Cancer 1991; 67: 2311–2326

11. Rijlaarsdam JU, Meijer CJLM, Willemze R. Differentiation between lymphadenosis benigna cutis and primary cutaneous follicular center cell lymphomas: a comparative clinicopathologic study of 57 patients. Cancer 1990; 65: 2301–2306

12. Cerroni L, Zöchling N, Pütz B, Kerl H. Detection of *Borrelia burgdorferi* in routinely-processed biopsy specimens of primary cutaneous B-cell lymphomas by PCR technique. J Cut Pathol 1997; 24: 457–461

13. Garbe C, Stein H, Dienemann D, Orfanos CE. *Borrelia burgdorferi*-associated cutaneous B cell lymphoma: clinical and immunohistologic characterization of four cases. J Am Acad Dermatol 1991; 24: 584–590

14. Wotherspoon AC, Ortiz-Hidalgo C, Falzon MR et al. *Helicobacter pylori*-associated gastritis and primary B-cell gastric lymphoma. Lancet 1991; 338: 1175–1176

15. Isaacson PG, Spencer J. Is gastric lymphoma an infectious disease? Hum Pathol 1993; 24: 569–570

16. Kerl H, Kresbach H. Germinal center cell-derived lymphomas of the skin. J Derm Surg Oncol 1984; 10: 291–295

17. Berti E, Alessi E, Caputo R et al. Reticulohistiocytoma of the dorsum. J Am Acad Dermatol 1988; 19: 259–272

18. Garcia CF, Weiss LM, Warnke RA, Wood GS. Cutaneous follicular lymphoma. Am J Surg Pathol 1986;10: 454–463

19. Cerroni L, Minkus G, Pütz B, Höfler H, Kerl H. Laser dissection of single lymphocytes and PCR-analysis in the diagnosis of cutaneous lymphoma. Br J Dermatol 1997; 136: 743–746

20. Willemze R, Meijer CJLM, Sentis HJ et al. Primary cutaneous large cell lymphomas of follicular center cell origin: a clinical follow-up study of 19 patients. J Am Acad Dermatol 1987; 16: 518–526

21. Dommann SN, Dommann-Scherrer CC, Zimmerman D et al. Primary cutaneous T-cell-rich B-cell lymphoma. A case report with a 13-year follow-up. Am J Dermatopathol 1995; 17: 618–624

22. Sander CA, Kaudewitz P, Kutzner H et al. T-cell-rich B-cell lymphoma presenting in skin. A clinicopathologic analysis of six cases. J Cut Pathol 1996; 23: 101–108

23. Cerroni L, Volkenandt M, Rieger E, Soyer HP, Kerl H. *bcl-2* protein expression and correlation with the interchromosomal 14;18 translocation in cutaneous lymphomas and pseudolymphomas. J Invest Dermatol 1994; 102: 231–235

24. Chimenti S, Cerroni L, Zenahlik P, Peris K, Kerl H. The role of MT2 and anti-bcl-2 protein antibodies in the differentiation of benign from malignant cutaneous infiltrates of B-lymphocytes with germinal center formation. J Cut Pathol 1996; 23: 319–322

25. Delia D, Borrello MG, Berti E et al. Clonal immunoglobulin gene rearrangements and normal T-cell receptor, bcl-2, and c-myc genes in primary cutaneous B-cell lymphomas. Cancer Res 1989; 49: 4901–4905

26. Bailey EM, Ferry JA, Harris NL et al. Marginal zone lymphoma (low-grade B-cell lymphoma of mucosa-associated lymphoid tissue type) of skin and subcutaneous tissue. A study of 15 patients. Am J Surg Pathol 1996; 20: 1011–1023

27. Rijlaarsdam JU, van der Putte SCJ, Berti E et al. Cutaneous immunocytomas: a clinicopathologic study of 26 cases. Histopathology 1993; 23: 117–125

28. Duncan LM, LeBoit PE. Are primary cutaneous immunocytoma and marginal zone lymphoma the same disease? Am J Surg Pathol 1997; 21: 1368–1372
29. LeBoit PE, McNutt NS, Reed JA, Jacobson M, Weiss LM. Primary cutaneous immunocytoma. A B-cell lymphoma that can easily be mistaken for cutaneous lymphoid hyperplasia. Am J Surg Pathol 1994; 18: 969–978
30. Torne R, Su WPD, Winkelmann RK, Smolle J, Kerl H. Clinicopathologic study of cutaneous plasmacytoma. Int J Dermatol 1990; 29: 562–566
31. Chang YT, Wong CK. Primary cutaneous plasmacytomas. Clin Exp Dermatol 1994; 19: 177–180
32. Wong KF, Chan JKC, Li LPK, Yau TK, Lee AWM. Primary cutaneous plasmacytoma. Report of two cases and review of the literature. Am J Dermatopathol 1994; 16: 392–397
33. Hurt MA, Santa Cruz DJ. Cutaneous inflammatory pseudotumor. Am J Surg Pathol 1990; 14: 764–773
34. Vermeer MH, Geelen FAMJ, van Haselen CW et al. Primary cutaneous large B-cell lymphomas of the legs. A distinct type of cutaneous B-cell lymphoma with an intermediate prognosis. Arch Dermatol 1996; 132: 1304–1308
35. Sheibani K, Battifora H, Winberg CD et al. Further evidence that 'malignant angioendotheliomatosis' is an angiotropic large-cell lymphoma. N Engl J Med 1986; 314: 943–948
36. Kutzner H, Englert W, Hellenbroich D et al. Angioendotheliomatosis proliferans systemisata: eine kutane Manifestation maligner B-Zellen-Lymphome – Histologische und immunohistochemische Untersuchungen an zwei Fällen. Hautarzt 1991; 42: 384–390
37. Sangueza O, Hyder DM, Sangueza P. Intravascular lymphomatosis: report of an unusual case with T cell phenotype occurring in an adolescent male. J Cut Pathol 1992; 19: 226–231
38. Perniciaro C, Winkelmann RK, Daoud MS, Su WPD. Malignant angioendotheliomatosis is an angiotropic lymphoma. Immunohistochemical, ultrastructural, and molecular genetic studies. Am J Dermatopathol 1995; 17: 242–248
39. Sander CA, Medeiros LJ, Abruzzo LV, Horak ID, Jaffe ES. Lymphoblastic lymphoma presenting in cutaneous sites: a clinicopathologic analysis of six cases. J Am Acad Dermatol 1991; 25: 1023–1031
40. Cerroni L, Zenahlik P, Kerl H. Specific infiltrates of B-cell chronic lymphocytic leukemia (B-CLL) arising at sites of herpes simplex and herpes zoster scars. Cancer 1995; 76: 26–31
41. Cerroni L, Zenahlik P, Höfler G et al. Specific cutaneous infiltrates of B-cell chronic lymphocytic leukemia. A clinicopathologic and prognostic study of 42 patients. Am J Surg Pathol 1996; 20: 1000–1010
42. Kerl H, Cerroni L. The morphologic spectrum of cutaneous B-cell lymphomas. Arch Dermatol 1996; 132: 1376–1377
43. Cerroni L, Gatter K, Kerl H. An Illustrated Guide to Skin Lymphoma. Oxford: Blackwell Science, 1998

2

Effects of light on skin

Deirdre Guerin

INTRODUCTION

Solar radiation is an important environmental hazard that can have many adverse effects on the skin, including acute sunburn, photosensitivity disorders, immunosuppression, photoageing and photocarcinogenesis.[1,2] The most damaging forms of light radiation to skin are ultravoilet A (UVA: 320–400 nm) and UVB (230–320 nm), although visible light and infrared can occasionally cause damage. The different wavelengths penetrate to different depths in the skin, and therefore cause damage at different levels (see Table 2.1). UVB causes more reactions in the epidermis, with only 10% reaching the dermis, whereas 50% of UVA reaches the dermis.[3]

Many substances in the skin can absorb UV light, including keratin proteins, haemoglobin, porphyrins, carotene, nucleic acids, melanin, lipoprotein, peptide bonds and aromatic amino acid residues including tryptophan, tyrosine and histidine.

When DNA absorbs UV light, covalent bonds are formed between adjacent thymidine molecules creating pyrimidine dimers. Cytidine dimers can also be

Table 2.1 Physical properties of light

Type of light	Wavelength	Type of skin damage
UVB	230 – 320 nm	Sunburn Non-melanoma skin cancer Photosensitivity disorders
UVA	320 – 400 nm	Photoageing Promotes UVB carcinogenicity Photosensitivity disorders
Visible light	400 – 760 nm	Photosensitivity disorders
Infrared	>760 nm	Can potentiate UV effects

Deirdre Guerin Consultant Pathologist, Department of Histopathology, Royal Liverpool University Hospital, Prescot Street, Liverpool L7 8XP

Table 2.2 Classification of light-related skin disorders

A. Genodermatoses
Xeroderma pigmentosum Cockayne's syndrome Bloom's syndrome Hartnup disease Rothmund Thomson disease

B. Metabolic/nutritional dermatoses
Porphyria Disorders of tryptophan metabolism Pellagra

C. Light sensitive dermatoses
Lupus erythematosus Lichen planus actinicus[6] Rosacea Hailey-Hailey disease Darier's disease Seborrhoeic dermatosis Atopic dermatosis Erythema multiforme Pityriasis rubra pilaris Disseminated superficial actinic porokeratosis Jessner's lymphocytic infiltrate

D. Photodermatoses	
Acute	*Chronic*
Phototoxic dermatitis Photoallergic dermatitis Hydroa vacciniforme Polymorphous light eruption Actinic prurigo Solar urticaria	Chronic actinic dermatitis/actinic reticuloid

formed.[4] Normal cells have several repair mechanisms to correct this, usually by excision repair.[5] If there is an abnormality in the DNA repair mechanism then cells with abnormal DNA persist and can lead to malignancy.

Light-related skin disorders can be classified into four groups as follows: genodermatoses, metabolic/nutritional disorders, light sensitive disorders and photodermatoses (see Table 2.2).

In this chapter, I will concentrate on the photodermatoses. These are a heterogeneous group of cutaneous disorders in which light plays a significant pathogenic role.

Most of these disorders are rare and they are dealt with in specialized photodermatology clinics. Histopathology may be used to diagnose one of these disorders, or to exclude malignancy in chronic photodermatoses. The following pages give a brief summary of the main features of these diseases, and hopefully provide a more complete picture of the similarities and differences between these difficult conditions.

PHOTODERMATOSES

PHOTOTOXIC DERMATITIS

This is the combination of ingestion of a photosensitizing substance and UV and/or visible radiation inducing damage. Phototoxicity may occur in up to 10.9% of patients treated with PUVA. An adverse effect may be found in 0.3% of treatments.[7]

Photosensitization is a process where there is an abnormal reaction to normally harmless radiation. This is induced by a photosensitizer, the ingestion or application of which causes another component (substrate) to be changed by the radiation.[4]

There is immediate involvement on exposure to sunlight. The patients develop erythema and an exaggerated sunburn reaction, which may blister or desquamate.

Histologically the damage may range from a few sunburn cells to epidermal necrosis.

Pseudoporphyria (see Table 2.3) is a type of phototoxic dermatitis that shows a clinical and histological similarity to porphyria cutanea tarda.[8] There is no abnormality of haem biosynthesis or of porphyrin excretion. The clinical features are bruising following minor trauma, erythema, vesicles and bullae on face, fingers and hands.[9]

PHOTOALLERGIC DERMATITIS

This is a delayed hypersensitivity reaction to the combination of topical photosensitizers (including substances found in fragrances and sunscreens) and UV radiation (see Table 2.4).

Table 2.3 Substances that can cause pseudoporphyria

Frusemide or thiazides in chronic renal failure
Naproxen and other Non-Steroidal Anti-Inflammatory Drugs (NSAIDs)
Dapsone
Tetracycline, doxycycline
Pyridoxine
Nalidixic acid
Vinblastine
Haemodialysis

NSAIDS = Non-Steroidal Anti-Inflammatory Drugs

Table 2.4 Substances that cause photoallergic dermatitis

Fragrance – musk ambrette
Coumarin
Sunscreen – hydroxybenzoates (parabens)
Benzophenones
Promethazine
Chlorpromazine
Tiaprofenic acid
Fentichlor
Carprofen
Anti-bacterial agents
Anti-microbial agents[10]
Pesticides[11]

The UV radiation alters an immunologically inactive molecule into an antigenic form. A reaction similar to allergic contact dermatitis is induced if the antigen stays in the skin or is formed subsequently. Pruritus and eczema start about 24 to 48 hours after exposure. The lesions may lichenify and spread beyond the light-exposed site. Lichenoid papules are especially seen when thiazide diuretics are being used. The lesions typically regress after 10–14 days. The disorder is more common in the elderly.[2] Histologically there is spongiosis and spongiotic vesiculation with exocytosis and a perivascular lymphocytic infiltrate. The skin may become acanthotic and develop focal parakeratosis. Rarely there can be a lichenoid reaction.

HYDROA VACCINIFORME

This is a rare debilitating photodermatosis of unknown aetiology that starts in childhood. Erythema and vesicles arise on sun-exposed sites 1–2 days after exposure and heal with scarring. It occurs in children starting at 3–5 years and recurs in spring and summer.[5] The differential diagnosis of porphyria is excluded by normal porphyrins.

Histologically, there are intraepidermal vesicles of serum and inflammatory cells. There is epidermal necrosis with ulceration and thrombosis.[12] In the dermis there is a perivascular lymphocytic and neutrophilic infiltrate,[13] and panniculitis may be seen in severe cases.

Direct immunofluorescence may show granular deposition of C3 at the dermoepidermal junction, but it is more often negative.[14]

The disease tends to improve spontaneously by puberty or early teenage years.[15]

If the eruption is related to latent Ebstein–Barr virus infection, there may be a relationship with lymphomatoid papulosis or lymphoma.[16]

HYDROA AESTIVALE

This is a mild form of hydroa vacciniforme. It has also been regarded as a childhood variant of polymorphous light eruption or a variant of erythropoietic protoporphyria.

JUVENILE SPRING ERUPTION

This is an epidemic papular photoeruption in children. The histology is similar to erythema multiforme.[15] It occurs in young boys in early spring and shows small papules and vesicles on the pinnae.[5]

POLYMORPHOUS LIGHT ERUPTION

Polymorphous light eruption (PLE) is a common acquired photodermatosis of unknown aetiology. It is a recurrent, delayed and transient abnormal cutaneous reaction to UV light.

PLE is thought to be a cell-mediated immune disease due to a delayed hypersensitivity response to an antigen induced by light exposure. However, no antigen has been identified.[13] Furthermore, 50% of cases are related to UVA exposure, 25% to UVB and 25% to a combination of UVA and UVB.[17] The initial reaction appears to be mediated by CD4+ cells, and a CD8+ infiltrate is present after about 72 hours. Langerhan's cells are also increased.[13]

PLE is most often seen in young white females, but does occur in other races.[18] There are no significant HLA types associated with polymorphous light eruption.[19]

Clinically there are non-scarring itchy erythematous plaques, papules and blisters on sun-exposed sites. The rash starts in spring and becomes less apparent as summer progresses. Lesions appear hours or days after exposure, and the duration of exposure is usually more than 30 minutes.[10] Lesions persist for days, and then resolve without scarring. Although there are six clinical subtypes, an individual patient tends to demonstrate one pattern only.

Histologically there is spongiosis, oedema of the papillary dermis and a perivascular chronic inflammatory cell infiltrate, composed mostly of T cells,[20] with a few histiocytes (Fig. 2.1).[21] Eosinophils and neutrophils may be seen.[22] There may be vesicles, parakeratosis and acanthosis.[23] The inflammation may extend into the deep dermis in established lesions.

Direct immunofluorescence may show some intervascular and perivascular fibrin deposition. IgM and C3 may be seen in venule walls. The clinical differen-

(A)

(B)

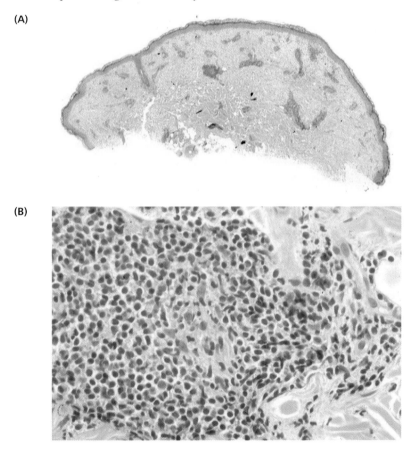

Fig. 2.1 Polymorphous light eruption. (**A**) This section shows skin with a prominent perivascular lymphocytic infiltrate. (**B**) Here, lymphocytic vasculitis is illustrated.

tial diagnosis includes lupus erythematosus (LE), drug reaction, solar urticaria and photosensitive erythema multiforme.[24] The histological differential diagnosis includes insect bite reaction, acute contact dermatitis, pityriasis lichenoides et varioliformis acuta and inflammatory pityriasis rosea.[22] Although LE patients are usually positive for autoantibodies, a small proportion (18%) of patients with PLE have low titres of autoantibodies, and these do not necessarily develop LE.[18,25] Also some subsets of LE patients demonstrate photosensitivity.

Usually PLE is self-limiting, although there is a slight increase in the incidence of autoimmune disorders (not LE).[26]

ACTINIC PRURIGO

This is a rare itchy papular rash that occurs in summer, usually on light exposed skin. Some 60% of cases are related to UVB exposure. Some authors regard it as a variant of polymorphous light eruption.

This is an idiopathic familial disorder seen more often in American Indians and Mexicans.[27,28] In South America, the disease is less seasonal, as there is more exposure to sunlight throughout the year.[29] No chromosomal abnormality has been reported.[30] There is a tenuous association with HLA-DR4,[31] A24 and Cw4.[32–34] However, this is complicated by the different HLA typing of the different races that are susceptible to this disease.[35]

Clinically there is a papular or nodular rash, which heals with pitted or linear scars. There is marked pruritus. The disorder may present early or late. Patients who develop the disease at a young age have a better prognosis.[28] In Mestizo populations in South America, signs of actinic prurigo appear in childhood.[36] Conjunctivitis and cheilitis may occur. Actinic prurigo can present clinically and histologically with acute or chronic lesions, and the patient may have both present at the same time.[32] The clinical differential diagnoses are with atopic eczema with photosensitivity,[28] chronic photocontact dermatitis and polymorphous light eruption.[36]

The histology of acute actinic prurigo is eczematous and non-specific.[21] There is excoriation, hyperkeratosis, parakeratosis, acanthosis, spongiosis, thickening of the basal lamina, perivascular lymphocytic infiltrate, endothelial cell swelling and red cell extravasation and vacuolar degeneration of basal keratinocytes. In chronic actinic prurigo, there is hyperkeratosis, acanthosis and elongation of the rete ridges.[32] There is also an eosinophilic variant.[37] Lesions on the lip may show large lymphoid germinal centres in the dermis.[32] Lip and conjunctival biopsies may be more specific than skin biopsies in the diagnosis of actinic prurigo.[38]

Immunofluorescence may be faintly positive in actinic prurigo but is usually negative in polymorphous light eruption.

SOLAR URTICARIA

This disorder may be caused by exposure to either visible light or UV light. It may be spontaneous or secondary to photosensitizing drugs or chemicals. The eruption starts within 5 minutes of exposure and resolves within hours.

The disorder is a Type 1 hypersensitivity reaction with circulating antibodies to IgE. There is also a rare fixed variant.[39] It usually begins between 20–40 years, persists indefinitely or gradually improves.[13]

Clinically there is burning and itching of exposed skin followed within a few minutes by patchy erythema and swelling (wheals). Occasionally there may be systemic manifestations including nausea, fainting and bronchospasm. There are six clinical subtypes, each due to a different wavelength.[40]

Histologically, there is dermal oedema and a mixed inflammatory cell infiltrate including neutrophils.

The differential diagnosis includes physical urticaria, porphyria, drug photosensitivity and lupus erythematosus.

CHRONIC ACTINIC DERMATITIS/ACTINIC RETICULOID

This is a chronic condition, which affects middle-aged and elderly male patients. Many have a long history of recurrent dermatitis of unknown cause. There is no seasonal variation and the rash may occur on sun-protected sites.

There are thick plaques and smooth papules on exposed skin, which may become confluent and resemble lymphoma. There may be generalized erythroderma. Shaded areas of the hands and face, such as skin creases, are often spared.

Chronic actinic dermatitis is due to abnormal photosensitivity to UVB and UVA with occasional extension into the visible light spectrum. Contact allergies to rubber components and fragrances are often present. The disorder is usually chronic, and improvement is only seen with avoidance of light. Pseudolymphomatoid chronic actinic dermatitis is known as actinic reticuloid.

Histologically, the appearances depend on the duration of the disease. In early lesions the features are rather non-specific. In later lesions, there are dense band-like lymphocytic infiltrates in the upper dermis, around vessels and adnexae and extending through the dermis to the subcutaneous fat (Fig. 2.2). There may be exocytosis, with the lymphocytes mimicking Pautrier microabscesses. Lymphocytes with large nuclei showing irregular nuclear outlines are frequent. Blast cells and mitotic figures are present. Dermal fibrosis is seen. Multinucleated stellate fibroblasts are present in the upper dermis.

There are conflicting reports of the CD4+/CD8+ ratio in this disease, although high levels of CD8+ cells are usually seen. There are dendritic cells expressing IgE in the dermal infiltrate. This feature has also been reported in atopic dermatitis. Elevated serum IgE may also be present.

The main differential diagnosis in the chronic phase is with mycosis fungoides. There are many features in common — the atypical lymphoid cells, the blast cells, the mitotic activity and the exocytosis. However, clinical features and investigation of UVA and UVB sensitivities should distinguish most cases.

PHOTOTESTING

The two main principles of phototesting are:

1. To provoke a reaction
2. To provoke a specific allergic response

(A)

(B)

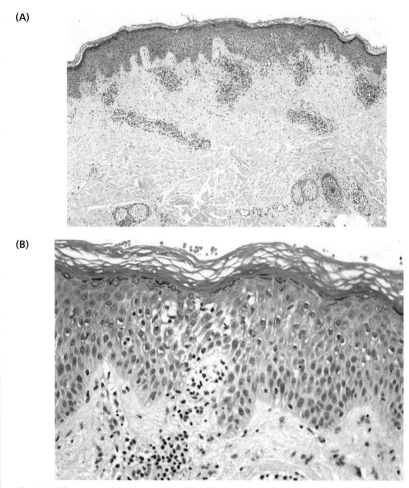

Fig. 2.2 Chronic actinic dermatitis. (**A**) This section shows a perivascular chronic inflammatory infiltrate in the upper dermis. (**B**) Here, exocytosis and groups of lymphocytes in the epidermis are illustrated.

MONOCHROMATOR TESTING

This is where a patient is exposed to light to provoke a response. It can be used to confirm that a disease is induced or exacerbated by light.

PHOTOALLERGY TESTING

This involves putting a photosensitizer on the skin and shining light of a specific wavelength on it. In this way, sensitivity to a particular waveband can be calculated. A control site using photosensitizer alone, without light, is used to exclude an allergic contact dermatitis.

The histology of a positive phototest shows occasional sunburn cells, spongiosis, exocytosis and a moderate perivascular chronic inflammatory cell infiltrate in the dermis.

KEY POINTS

1. Solar radiation can have many adverse effects on the skin that can be classified into four groups: genodermatoses, metabolic/nutritional disorders, light sensitive disorders and photodermatoses.
2. Only the photodermatoses were considered in this chapter. They are a heterogeneous group in which light plays a significant pathogenic role.
3. There are six acute photodermatoses, which were briefly summarized giving details of symptoms and histology.
4. The single chronic photodermatoses, chronic actinic dermatitis/actinic reticuloid, was also described and details of different diagnosis given.

REFERENCES

1. Abel EA, Deneau DG, Farber EM, Price NM, Hoppe RT. PUVA treatment of erythrodermic and plaque type mycosis fungoides. J Am Acad Dermatol 1981; 4: 423–429
2. Hawk JLM. Photosensitivity in the elderly. Br J Dermatol 1990; 122s35: 29–41
3. Rhodes LE. Topical and systemic approaches for protection against solar radiation-induced skin damage. Clin Dermatol 1998; 16: 75–82
4. Ramsay CA. Photosensitivity in children. Ped Clin N Am 1983; 30: 687–699
5. Isaacson D, Turner ML, Elgart ML. Summertime actinic lichenoid eruption (lichen planus actinicus). J Am Acad Dermatol 1981; 4: 404–411
6. Morison WL, Marwaha S, Beck L. PUVA-induced phototoxicity: incidence and causes. J Am Acad Dermatol 1997; 36: 183–185
7. Gonzalez E, Gonzalez S. Drug photosensitivity, idiopathic photodermatoses and sunscreens. J Am Acad Dermatol 1996; 35: 871–885
8. Poh-Fitzpatrick M. Porphyria, pseudoporphyria, pseudopseudoporphyria? Arch Dermatol 1986; 122: 403–404
9. Harber LC, Bickers DR. Porphyria and pseudoporphyria. J Invest Dermatol 1984; 82: 207–209
10. Fotiades J, Soter NA, Lim HW. Results of evaluation of 203 patients for photosensitivity in a 7.3 year period. J Am Acad Dermatol 1995; 33: 597–602
11. Mark KA, Brancaccio RR, Soter NA, Cohen DE. Allergic contact and photoallergic contact dermatitis to plant and pesticide allergens. Arch Dermatol 1999; 135: 67–70
12. Sonnex TS, Hawk JLM. Hydroa vacciniforme: a review of ten cases. Br J Dermatol 1988; 118: 101–108
13. Norris PG, Hawk JLM. The acute idiopathic photodermatoses. Sem Dermatol 1990; 9: 32–38
14. Goldgeier MH, Nordlund JJ, Lucky AW et al. Hydroa vacciniforme. Arch Dermatol 1982; 118: 588–591
15. Halasz CL, Leach EE, Walther RR, Poh-Fitzpatrick MB. Hydroa vacciniforme: induction of lesions with ultraviolet A. J Am Acad Dermatol 1983; 8: 171–176
16. Iwatsuki K, Xu Z, Takata M et al. The association of latent Epstein-Barr virus infection with hydroa vacciniforme. Br J Dermatol 1999; 140: 715–721
17. Ortel B, Tanew A, Wolff K, Honigsmann H. Polymorphous light eruption: action spectrum and photoprotection. J Am Acad Dermatol 1986; 14: 748–753
18. Mastalier U, Kerl H, Wolf P. Clinical, laboratory, phototest and phototherapy findings in polymorphic light eruption: a retrospective study of 133 patients. Eur J Dermatol 1998; 8: 554–559
19. Lane PR, Sheridan DP, Hogan DJ, Moreland A. HLA typing in polymorphous light eruption. J Am Acad Dermatol 1991; 24: 570–573
20. Moncada B, Gonzalez-Amaro R, Baranda ML, Loerdo C, Urbina R. J Am Acad Dermatol 1984; 10: 970–973
21. Grabczynska SA, McGregor JM, Hawk JLM, Calonje E. Histological spectrum of actinic prurigo and polymorphic light eruption. Br J Dermatol 1997; 137s50: 62 (Abstract)

22. Hood AF, Elpern DJ, Morison WL. Histopathologic findings in papulovesicular light eruption. J Cut Path 1986; 13: 13–21

23. Epstein JH. Polymorphous light eruption. J Am Acad Dermatol 1980; 3: 329–343

24. Holzle E, Plewig G, von Kries R, Lehmann P. Polymorphous light eruption. J Invest Dermatol 1987; 88: 32s–38s

25. Kiss M, Husz S, Dobozy A. The occurrence of antinuclear, anti-SSA/Ro and anti-SSB/La antibodies in patients with polymorphous light eruption. Acta Dermatol Venereol (Stockh) 1991; 71: 341–343

26. Hasan T, Ranki A, Jansen CT, Karvonen J. Disease associations in polymorphous light eruption. Arch Dermatol 1998; 134: 1081–1085

27. Magana M. Actinic or solar prurigo. J Am Acad Dermatol 1997; 35: 504–505

28. Lane PR, Hogan DJ, Martel MJ, Reeder B, Irvine J. Actinic prurigo: clinical features and prognosis. J Am Acad Dermatol 1992; 26: 683–692

29. Lane PR. Actinic prurigo. Int J Dermatol 1995; 34(5): 363–364

30. Scheen SR, Connolly SM, Dicken CH. Actinic prurigo. J Am Acad Dermatol 1980; 5: 183–190

31. Dawe RS, Collins P, Ferguson J, O'Sullivan A. Actinic prurigo and HLA-DR4. J Invest Dermatol 1997; 108: 233–234

32. Lane PR, Murphy F, Hogan DJ, Hull PR, Burgdorf WHC. Histopathology of actinic prurigo. Am J Dermatol 1993: 15: 326–331

33. Hojyo-Tomoka T, Granados J, Vargas-Alarcon G et al. Further evidence of the role of HLA-DR4 in the genetic susceptibility to actinic prurigo. J Am Acad Dermatol 1997; 36: 935–937

34. Bernal JE, Duran de Rueda MM, de Brigard S. Human lymphocyte antigen in actinic prurigo. J Am Acad Dermatol 1988; 18: 310–312

35. Sheridan DP, Lane PR, Irvine J, Martel M, Hogan DJ. HLA typing in actinic prurigo. J Am Acad Dermatol 1990; 22: 1019–1023

36. Hojyo-Tomoka T, Vega-Memije E, Granados J et al. Actinic prurigo: an update. Int J Dermatol 1995; 34: 380–384

37. Grabczynska SA, Roberts NM, McGregor JM, Hawk JLM. An unusual photodermatosis – a case for diagnosis. Presented at: The Royal Society of Medicine, Section of Dermatology, April 1999

38. Hojyo-Tomoka T, Vega E, Romero A, Reyes M, Carrasoo D. Actinic prurigo. Int J Dermatol 1992; 31: 372–373

39. Reinauer S, Leenutaphong V, Holzle E. Fixed solar urticaria. J Am Acad Dermatol 1993; 29: 161–165

40. Thiers BH, Dobson RL. Westwood conference on clinical dermatology. J Am Acad Dermatol 1981; 4: 487–494

41. Toonstra J. Actinic reticuloid. Sem Diag Pathol 1991; 8: 109–116

3

Reactive and neoplastic histiocytic skin disorders

Janine Wechsler

Histiocytic disorders are the result of either reactive hyperplasia or neoplastic proliferation of histiocytes.[1-4] The role of histiocytes in phagocytosis and antigen presentation explains why they are implicated in many pathological processes affecting the skin, which represents a zone of exchange between the body and the external environment.

CHARACTERISTICS OF HISTIOCYTES

During recent years there have been considerable changes in our understanding of the concept of the histiocyte/macrophage system.[5] All categories of histiocytes are derived from the bone marrow by multiplication from a stem cell. The derived cells migrate from the bone marrow to the blood as monocytes. They circulate through the body and stop in various organs where they differentiate into histiocytes, which form part of the mononuclear phagocyte system (MPS).[5] Histiocytes have some common morphological and phenotypical features. Their cytoplasm is eosinophilic and contains variable amounts of lysosomes. They bear the membrane receptor Fc for IgG and the fragment C3 of complement. They express the common leucocyte antigens CD45, CD14, CD33, class HLA I (A,B,C), class HLA II (DP, DQ, DR) and CD4. ATPasic and esterasic membrane enzymatic markers have also been demonstrated. Histiocytes are actively involved in the immune response by way of two distinct functions: phagocytic activity and antigen presentation. Extensive immunological studies have demonstrated a dichotomy for these two functions. Phagocytic activity is the main property of the macrophages, while antigen presentation is restricted to non- or poorly phagocytic cells, referred to as dendritic cells because of their star-like appearance.[6] Macrophages and dendritic cells are derived from a common bone marrow progenitor that has undergone different differentiation processes under the influence of environmental factors and various growth factors such as granulocyte-

Janine Wechsler MD, Département de Pathologie, Hôpital Henri Mondor, Université, Paris-Val-de-Marne, 94010 Créteil, France

macrophage colony-stimulating factor (GM-CSF),[7,8] tumor necrosis factor-alpha (TNF-α),[8] or interleukin-4 (IL-4).[9] The various categories of histiocytes are distinguishable on the basis of their morphology, phenotype and function.

Macrophages are highly variable in morphology and size. Their cytoplasm contains numerous lysosomes in relation to their phagocytic activity. They express the KiM1p antigen, which belongs to the CD68 marker family. Intracytoplasmic enzymes include esterase and lysozyme.

Dendritic cells have an indented nucleus and cytoplasm with thin dendritic processes. Their main activity is antigen presentation, which represents a necessary step during the initiation of the immune response. In addition they express Factor XIIIa, CD1c and class II HLA antigens.[10]

A subset of dendritic cells differentiates into Langerhans cells (LCs) after an indeterminate stage of differentiation.[11] This maturation occurs in squamous epithelium, lymph nodes, spleen and bronchiolar epithelium. The anatomical location of dendritic cells facilitates their contact with antigens, which they then bear and fix to class II HLA antigens before presenting them to lymphocytes by means of their cytoplasmic processes. They also bear Fc and C3 receptors.[12] The demonstration by Murphy et al[13] that epidermal LCs bear the CD1a antigen, normally present on the surface of thymocytes, marked a crucial step in our understanding of LCs. They also express S-100 protein.[14] Their cytoplasm contains zipper-like inclusions named Birbeck granules, measuring from 190 to 360 nm in length and 33 nm in width. More than 30 years after their first description, the origin of these structures is still controversial.[15] Normally, histiocytes do not proliferate in tissues, but some factors can induce histiocytic hyperplasia. Benign and malignant histiocytic neoplasias of unknown aetiology may also occur.

PATHOLOGICAL IMPLICATIONS OF HISTIOCYTES

REACTIVE HISTIOCYTIC HYPERPLASIAS

Reactive hyperplasias are more common than neoplastic proliferations of histiocytes.[16] Factors such as infections, foreign body reactions, degeneration of connective tissue and even neoplastic disorders induce reactive histiocytic hyperplasias, which may involve each of the three families of histiocytes. For instance, mycobacterial infections are known to induce macrophagic epithelioid granulomas, necrobiosis lipoidica, granuloma annulare and necrobiotic xanthogranuloma.[17] Other degenerative changes in collagen provoke a peripheral histiocytic reaction (Fig. 3.1). Macrophagic granulomas are found in distinct variants of cutaneous T-cell lymphomas.[18,19]

Haemophagocytic or erythrophagocytic lymphohistiocytosis belongs to a group of reactive histiocytic disorders that may be familial or sporadic. Epstein–Barr virus (EBV) infection may induce such a process. The major diagnostic criteria are fever, splenomegaly, cytopaenia, hypofibrinogenaemia and haemophagocytosis. Non-specific rashes with infiltrates of lymphocytes and activated histiocytes are found in 10% of cases.[20]

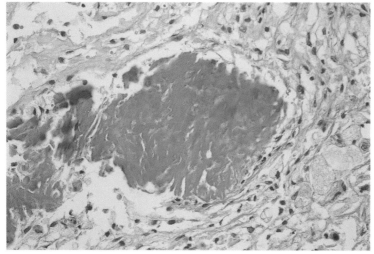

Fig. 3.1 Reactive histiocytic reaction in necrobiotic xanthogranuloma: accumulation of clear foamy histiocytes at the periphery of an area of degenerative connective tissue. (haematoxylin & eosin: × 200.)

HISTIOCYTOSES

Histiocytoses are due to the neoplastic proliferation of histiocytes. They are a group of heterogeneous conditions, some of which correspond to congenital syndromes.[21] They have been grouped on the basis of their morphological features. Unlike the reactive hyperplasias, the mechanisms provoking neoplastic proliferation of histiocytes are still unknown: an excessive immune reaction to a viral infection has been suggested but not confirmed.[22,23] Recently a monoclonal proliferation of histiocytes has been demonstrated in cases of Langerhans' cell histiocytosis.[24,25]

However, with increasing understanding of the biology of histiocytes, more rational terminology and classification systems have appeared. In 1985, the *Histiocyte Society* proposed a new classification of histiocytoses in which Langerhans' cell histiocytoses form class I, non-Langerhans' cell histiocytoses form class II and malignant histiocytoses form class III.[26]

More recently, the WHO Committee on histiocytic/reticulum cell proliferations has proposed a classification based on the presumed lineage of lesional cells: LC, indeterminate cell, dendrocyte and macrophage lineage (Table 3.1).[27]

LANGERHANS' CELL HISTIOCYTOSES (CLASS I HISTIOCYTOSES)

Light microscopy shows the accumulation of large histiocytes with eosinophilic cytoplasm and lobulated or reniform nuclei (Fig. 3.2). These cells are associated with lymphocytes and eosinophils. In long-standing lesions fibrosis is observed; xanthomatization and a granulomatous reaction may occur.[28,29]

Like normal LCs, neoplastic cells in LC histiocytosis express S-100 protein and CD1a antigen (Fig. 3.3), which can be demonstrated in frozen sections as well as in fixed material.[30] On electron microscopy they contain Birbeck granules. Some differences between normal and neoplastic LCs have been stressed.[31-34] The expression of the interleukin 2 receptor, immunoreactivity with peanut

Table 3.1 Classification of histiocytoses according to their presumed cell lineage

Presumed lineage	Histiocytosis
Langerhans' cell	Histiocytosis X Congenital self-healing reticulohistiocytosis
Indeterminate cell	Indeterminate cell histiocytoma/histiocytosis Generalized eruptive histiocytoma Benign cephalic histiocytosis
Dendrocyte	Disseminated dermal dendrocytoma Xanthoma disseminatum Juvenile/adult xanthogranuloma Reticulohistiocytoma cutis Multicentric reticulohistiocytosis Necrobiotic xanthogranuloma Progressive nodular histiocytosis Hereditary progressive mucinous histiocytosis Familial histiocytic dermoarthritis Erdheim–Chester disease
Macrophage	Haemophagocytic syndromes Sinus histiocytosis of Rosai–Dorfman

Source: Wood & Haber 1993.[27]

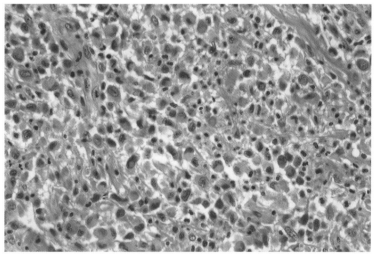

Fig. 3.2 Eosinophilic granuloma, a variant of Langerhans' cell histiocytosis exhibiting an accumulation of mononuclear cells with reniform nucleus, mixed with numerous eosinophils. (haematoxylin & eosin: × 200.)

agglutinin and antibodies to interferon gamma, as well as diminished antigen-presenting function, suggest that the pathological cells in LC histiocytosis are abnormal LCs or at least cells in an altered state of activation.[31]

Langerhans' cell histiocytoses were previously regrouped into the so-called histiocytosis X.[33] Whether it is accurate to distinguish the three forms: Letterer–Siwe disease, Hand–Schüller–Christian disease and eosinophilic granuloma is still debated. These three conditions have a similar histopathological pattern, and cross-over forms may occur. For these reasons some authors prefer the terms: acute, progressive and localized forms of Langerhans' cell histiocytosis.[3,35] The

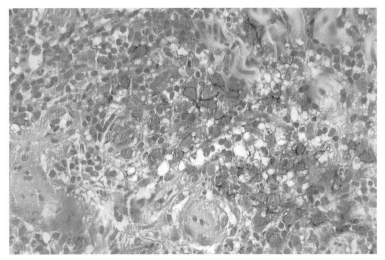

Fig. 3.3 Eosinophilic granuloma. Histiocytes are CD1a-positive. (Immunophosphatasic method: × 200.)

general tendency now is to distinguish benign and malignant subgroups. However the recent discovery of a monoclonal proliferation in variants of LC histiocytosis with differing prognoses makes this distinction questionable.

The benign subgroup of Langerhans' cell histiocytoses includes the following:

1. Eosinophilic granuloma. This is usually a localized osseous lesion in children or young adults (15–30 years). Cutaneous nodules may occur, especially in periorificial areas.
2. Congenital self-healing reticulohistiocytosis (Hashimoto–Pritzker's disease). In this entity, lesions are exclusively cutaneous. They do not affect mucosal membranes. They are made up of multiple and disseminated ulcerative papules and nodules that often exist at birth. The lesions regress within several months. However close clinical follow-up is recommended because some rare cases may evolve into another form of LC histiocytosis.[36]
3. Hand–Schüller–Christian syndrome. This disease occurs in children and young adults. It is typically associated with osteolytic lesions in flat bones, diabetes insipidus and exophthalmos. In fact, this triad is rarely found (17% according to Oberman).[37] Osteolytic lesions are the most frequent, being present in 80% of cases, diabetes insipidus in 50% and exophthalmos in 10–30%. Cutaneous lesions occur in 30% of the cases. There is an increasing number of CD68-positive macrophages in ageing lesions.[15] Partial xanthomatization of these macrophages may be responsible for confusion with juvenile xanthogranulomas. CD1a-positive nests of mononuclear round-shaped histiocytes and epidermotropism are clues for the diagnosis of LC histiocytosis.

The course of the disease is characterized by either spontaneous regression or multivisceral dissemination with poor prognosis. Studying 14 cases of Langerhans' cell histiocytosis with skin involvement, Geissman et al[38] demonstrated that lack of expression of E-cadherin was associated with extracutaneous dissemination of LC histiocytosis.

The association of LC histiocytosis with another malignant neoplasm appears to be more frequent than in the general population. Evaluation of 54 patients detected two patterns of association: first, the secondary neoplasia may be promoted by therapy-induced immunosuppression; second, a genetic predisposition with or without immunosuppression.[39]

1. Letterer–Siwe disease. This systemic disease occurs in 6-month-old to 2-year-old children. Muco-cutaneous lesions are present in 50% of the cases. Patients exhibit translucent papules and/or seborrheic keratoses.[40] The neoplastic CD1a-positive histiocytes predominate in the superficial dermis and show frequent epidermotropism. They are mixed with eosinophils. Cutaneous involvement is not necessarily a benign feature and many patients progress to multi-system disease.[41]

2. Malignant histiocytosis X or interdigitated-cell sarcoma. This entity is very rare. Only a few cases have been reported. Patients exhibit an aggressive disease with visceral involvement and rapidly fatal outcome.[42]

NON-LANGERHANS' CELL HISTIOCYTOSES (CLASS II HISTIOCYTOSES)

Zelger et al[43] presented a unifying concept for this heterogeneous group of non-LC histiocytoses. They emphasized the fact that the common denominator of these histiocytoses is the presence of KiM1p-positive monocyte/macrophage-derived cells. On the basis of the cytological appearance, they described five types of mononuclear histiocytes (Fig. 3.4): (i) vacuolated cells with round to oval nuclei and ill-defined clear cytoplasm; (ii) xanthomatized cells with well-demarcated cytoplasm containing tiny vacuoles; (iii) scalloped cells with angulated cytoplasm; (iv) oncocytic cells with ground-glassy eosinophilic cytoplasm; (v) spindle shaped cells. Three multinucleate cell types were also defined: xanthomatized (Touton), oncocytic and foreign-body-type giant cells. According to this unifying concept, the authors stipulated that the composition of these cell types

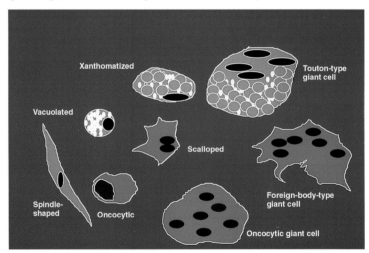

Fig. 3.4 Diagram of the cytological types of non-Langerhans' cell histiocytoses, according to the unifying concept proposed by Zelger et al[43] for classifying such non-LC histiocytoses. Five types of mononuclear histiocytes were described: vacuolated, xantomatized, scalloped, oncocytic and spindle-shaped. Three multinucleate cell types were also defined: xanthomatized (Touton cells), oncocytic and foreign-body-type giant cells.

Table 3.2 Unifying concept for non-Langerhans' cell histiocytoses according to Zelger

Predominant cell type	Localized forms	Generalized forms	Association with internal diseases
Various cell types	Juvenile and adult XG		No
Vacuolated	Monomorphous variant of XG		No
	Benign cephalic H		No
		Generalized eruptive histiocytoma	No
	Solitary indeterminate cell histiocytoma		No
		Indeterminate cell H	Acute mast cell leukemia
Xanthomatized	Solitary papular xanthoma	Generalized papular xanthomas	Diabetes insipides; myeloma
		Xanthoma disseminatum	Systemic involvement[65]
		Erdheim–Chester disease	No
	Cutaneous sinus H	Sinus H of Rosai–Dorfman	Massive lymphadenopathy
			Polyclonal gammapathy
Scalloped	Monomorphous variant of adult XG		No
Oncocytic	Reticulohistiocytoma cutis		No
		Multicentric reticulohistiocytosis	Arthropathy. Internal malignancy[49]
Spindle cell	Monomorphous variant of juvenile XG		No
		Progressive nodular H	No
		Hereditary progressive mucinous H	No

Abbreviations used: H, histiocytosis; XG, xanthogranuloma; Sd, syndrome.
Source: Zelger et al 1996.[43]

lead to different diagnoses 'which, interestingly, favour certain clinical settings' (Table 3.2).

Polymorphous type

Juvenile and adult xanthogranuloma (XG)[43-45] is characterized by a broad spectrum of various types of histiocytes. Within the histiocytic component, which usually comprises 95% of the infiltrate, mononuclear to multinuclear variants are observed (Fig. 3.5). The most numerous are mononuclear cells. Vacuolated, xanthomatized (Fig. 3.6) and spindle-shaped (Fig. 3.7) cells predominate in juvenile XG, whereas scalloped and oncocytic cells predominate in adult XG. The spindle cell variant is an early stage of XG in children (Fig. 3.6). In addition to mononuclear cells, multinucleate giant cells are present in variable numbers. The

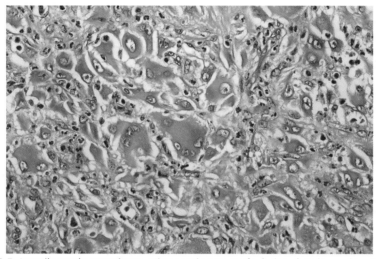

Fig. 3.5 Juvenile xanthogranuloma. Microscopic aspect of a lesion showing various types of mononuclear to multinuclear histiocytes mixed with lymphocytic infiltrate. (haematoxylin & eosin: × 200).

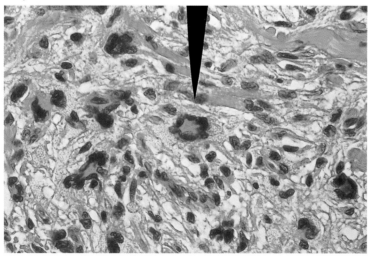

Fig. 3.6 Xanthomatized variant of juvenile XG. Xanthomatized cells with typical multinucleate Touton cells. (haematoxylin & eosin × 400.)

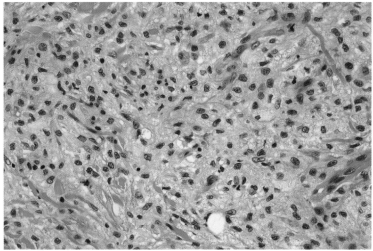

Fig. 3.7 Spindle cell variant of juvenile XG. This form, occurring in children, may mimic a fibroblastic tumor. (haematoxylin & eosin: × 200.)

histiocytic component is associated with mixed infiltrates of small lymphocytes, plasma cells, neutrophils and eosinophils.

Predominantly xanthomatized type

All variants of xanthomas are made of xanthomatized cells accumulated in the dermis. These mononuclear cells are mixed with multinucleated giant Touton cells. According to the clinical presentation, and the association with other conditions, xanthomatized type entities are classified into distinct categories.[40,43]

- Xanthomas and xanthelasmas associated with dyslipidæmia are storage diseases, but not proliferative disorders. Skin biopsy is usually not necessary to establish the diagnosis.
- Papular xanthomas. Lesions consist of multiple muco-cutaneous papules that are yellow and non-confluent. Blood lipid levels are normal. Spontaneous regression of the lesions may occur.[46]
- Xanthoma disseminatum (XD) is a rare and usually benign condition involving skin and mucous membranes in young men. Clinically, the lesions are reddish papules, nodules or confluent plaques. They are bilateral and symmetrical, predominantly located on the face, the trunk and the flexures. Ocular mucosae and pituitary gland may also be infiltrated. Diabetes insipidus is present in 50% of cases. Some reports have provided evidence of an association between XD and multiple myeloma.[47,48]

Predominantly oncocytic type

- Multicentric reticulohistiocytosis is a rare condition predominantly occuring in young females in which multiple erythematous skin nodules are associated with a destructive arthropathy. An association with an internal malignancy was reported in 28% of the patients studied.[49] Reticulohistiocytoma cutis is the benign solitary variant of multicentric reticulohistiocytosis.[50] Cutaneous infiltrates are rich in multinucleate oncocytic histiocytes with a large ground-

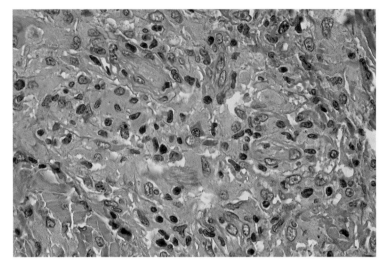

Fig. 3.8 Multicentric reticulohistiocytosis. Dermal infiltration of oncocytic histiocytes with a large ground-glassy cytoplasm. (haematoxylin & eosin × 200.)

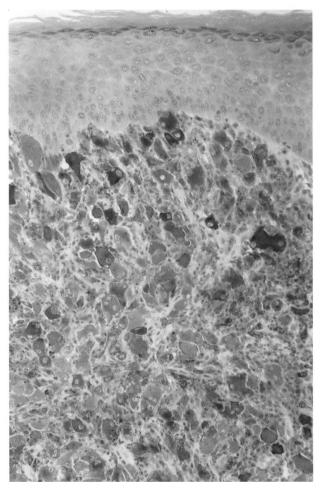

Fig. 3.9 Multicentric reticulohistiocytosis. The cells that infiltrate the dermis are strongly stained by macrophagic markers, herein anti-KP1. (Immunophosphatasic method: × 400.)

glassy cytoplasm containing numerous PAS-positive inclusions (Fig. 3.8). The cells are strongly stained by macrophagic markers such as anti-CD68 (Fig. 3.9)

Predominantly vacuolated type

- Benign cephalic histiocytosis[51] occurs on the head and neck in children in the first year of life. The clinical presentation is of a papular eruption. Papules are 2–3 mm in size and erythematous to yellowish in colour. Histologically it is a monomorphous vacuolated variant of XG. The lesions usually regress after 2–5 years.
- Generalized eruptive histiocytosis. This disease occurs in adults and presents with symmetrical red-brown papules.[52] Mucosal lesions may be present. All the signs usually regress within a few years. This condition is probably similar, if not identical, to benign cephalic histiocytosis, which may represent a regional variant of the same disease. In addition, some reports on cases of generalized eruptive histiocytosis suggest overlap between these cases and indeterminate cell histiocytosis.[27]

Predominantly spindle-cell type

- Spindle-cell variant of XG (mentioned above) is a pecular form of XG in children.[43]
- Nodular progressive histiocytosis. Patients present with confluent papules on the face that progress to develop a 'leonine' appearance. There is no mucosal lesion.[40] In addition to the spindle-shaped histiocytes, the dermal infiltrate contains lymphocytes. The lesions do not regress spontaneously.
- Hereditary progressive mucinous histiocytosis. This is a recently described entity which is a rare autosomal dominant histiocytosis. Patients have a progressive eruption of skin-coloured to red-brown papules distributed on the face and limbs. Nodular agregates of epithelioid and tightly packed spindle cells are seen in the mid dermis. These cells are dendrocytes that are Factor XIIIa positive, S-100 and CD1a negative.[53]
- Familial sea-blue histiocytosis. Zina et al[54] reported a case of this rare autosomal recessive disorder with skin involvement that was characterized by disseminated infiltration of unusual macrophages containing granules that appeared to be blue-green with a Giemsa stain and to have rod-like cytoplasmic inclusions on electronic microscopy.

NON-LANGERHANS' CELL HISTIOCYTOSIS OF UNKNOWN CELL LINEAGE

- Indeterminate cell histiocytosis. This is a clinicopathological entity with features of both X and non-X histiocytosis.[55,56] It has been rarely reported in the literature. The indeterminate cells have been considered to be the precursors of the epidermal–dermal dendritic cell system.[57-59]
- Sinus histiocytosis with massive lymphadenopathy or Rosai–Dorfman disease. This rare condition combines features of Langerhans' and non-Langerhans' cell histiocytoses. It usually involves cervical nodes in children. Rare cases of skin-limited disease were reported as cutaneous sinus histiocytosis (CSH).[60] There is a dense infiltrate in the dermis, which is composed mainly of large histiocytes mixed with lymphocytes, plasma cells, neutrophils and erythrocytes. Intact-appearing ingested cells are seen within

intra-cytoplasmic vacuoles of the histiocytes, which show emperipolesis (Fig. 3.10). The nature of the CSH cells is still a matter of debate. In the skin, they have been reported to express CD1a[61] and S-100 protein[60,61] as LCs (Fig. 3.11), and Factor XIIIa[61] as dendrocytes. Patients with CSH have only a low risk of developing systemic disease.

- Erdheim–Chester disease (ECD). ECD is a rare condition occurring in adults. Tissue infiltration by foamy histiocytes (Fig. 3.12) and symmetrical osteosclerosis of long bones are the main features of this disease. Although bone involvement is invariably present, ECD can present as a systemic condition with life-threatening visceral involvement.[62,63] Skin lesions can occur as xanthomas.[64,65] In spite of their many differences, ECD and LC histiocytosis seem to be related entities. Patients with both conditions have been reported.[65] Such

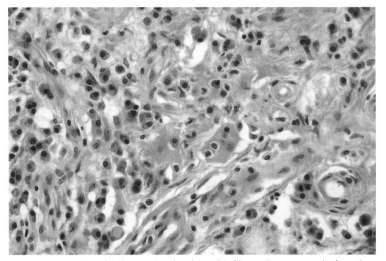

Fig. 3.10 Cutaneous sinus histiocytosis. The dermal infiltrate is composed of a mixture of lymphocytes, plasma cells, neutrophils and erythrocytes. Intact-appearing ingested cells are seen within intra-cytoplasmic vacuoles of the histiocytes that show emperipolesis. (haematoxylin & eosin: × 200.)

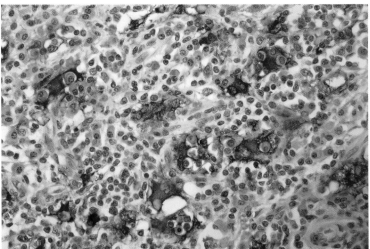

Fig. 3.11 Cutaneous sinus histiocytosis. Giant cells express S-100 protein. (Immunophosphatasic method: × 400.)

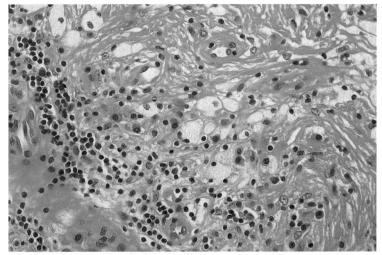

Fig. 3.12 Erdheim–Chester disease. The cellular infiltration is composed of a polymorphous infiltrate containing large foamy histiocytes mixed with plasma cells, lymphocytes and fibrosis. There is no atypia. (haematoxylin & eosin: × 200.)

cases are informative. Both LCs and ECD histiocytes are derived from bone marrow stem cells, with differentiation into dendritic/LCs in the former and a supposed differentiation into the mononuclear phagocytic system in the latter.[3] However an explanation for the occurence of both entities concomitantly could be that histiocytes deriving from the mononuclear phagocytic system might further differentiate into LCs.[15]

MALIGNANT HISTIOCYTOSES AND TRUE HISTIOCYTIC LYMPHOMA

The improvement of immunohistochemical techniques has led to a reclassification of many cases previously supposed to be of histiocytic origin into B or T-cell lymphomas.[66] Nevertheless, a small number of cases show characteristics of monocytic–macrophage proliferation.[67] In order to be considered as true histiocytic lymphomas such tumours must be demonstrated to be CD68–positive.

DIFFICULTIES IN DIAGNOSIS AND CLASSIFICATION

Several facts may explain the difficulties in diagnosis and classification of histiocytoses. The identification of histiocytes are based on microscopy, ultrastructural morphology and immunophenotype. Except for LC histiocytosis, molecular biological results are not yet available in this field of pathology. Moreover, variations and discrepancies in immunohistochemical and ultrastructural data may be due to technical variation and type of tissue processing used (nitrogen frozen material, variable fixatives, antibody concentrations, micro-wave procedure duration etc).

Some entities such as sinus histiocytosis with massive lymphadenopathy, ECD and indeterminate cell histiocytosis, exhibit features of both LC and non-LC histiocytoses.

Histiocytes expressing distinct phenotypes can be found in the same tumour. For instance in lesions of LC histiocytosis, it is possible to find groups or single units of CD68-positive cells in addition to CD1a-positive LCs.[15,68] It is difficult, therefore, to know whether this finding is due to the mixture of two distinct populations, LCs and macrophages, or is related to a different stage of maturation of cells that belong to the same lineage.[59] The hypothesis that an incomplete phenotype might reflect an early stage of maturation was supported by investigative studies on cultures of dendrocytes.[6] Moreover, it is possible that histiocytic populations show variations due to the time course of the lesions.[9] Also one cannot exclude the possibility that some neoplastic histiocytes could bear an abnormal phenotype.

With regard to the differential diagnosis, the distinction between the monomorphous spindle-cell variant of xanthogranulomas or progressive nodular histiocytosis from dermatofibromas may be problematic. A storiform pattern is usually present in dermatofibromas, which is not found in the former disease. If present, xanthomization is limited to small foci of cells in dermatofibromas whereas it is diffuse in papular xanthomas. The major problems are raised by some rare variants of dermatofibromas such as epithelioid cell histiocytoma and clear cell dermatofibroma, which may mimic the scalloped and vacuolated variants of non-LC histiocytoses, respectively. Clinically dermatofibromas occur on the legs in women; histologically some of the following features may be present and would favour the diagnosis of dermatofibroma: epidermal hyperplasia, polypoid shape with a collarette formation, storiform pattern, ectasic vessels, monster-like giant cells, prominent iron deposition.

A giant cell or oncocytic histiocytic response is seen in foreign-body reactions, necrobiotic xanthogranuloma, necrobiosis lipoidica and granuloma annulare, which are examples of histiocytic disorders that are due to collagen or ground substance degeneration, as was mentioned above.

KEY POINTS

1. The classification of histiocytoses into Langerhans' and non-Langerhans' cell histiocytoses is now well agreed.
2. The unifying term Langerhans' cell histiocytosis is favoured over the term histiocytosis X. In spite of biological advances especially with the demonstration of the clonality of some LCs proliferations, the causal factors of the disease are still largely unknown.
3. Non-Langerhans' cell histiocytoses form a heterogeneous and often confusing group of entities. One reason for the difficulties in classifying these histiocytoses is that the monocyte–macrophage system is composed of dynamic cells that are able to change in morphology, immunophenotype and functional state, depending on environmental factors.
4. The unifying concept proposed by Zelger et al[43] is a tentative attempt at simplifying the understanding of non-LC histiocytoses. It is important to note that this method of classification which is based upon the cytological appearance of the histiocytic cells, is able to determine clinico-pathological correlation in a number of these entities.
5. In the future, advances in understanding of the biology of the so-called 'mononuclear phagocytic and immunoregulatory effector system' will provide the basis for the development of more rational classification systems.

REFERENCES

1. Basset F, Nezelof C, Hance AJ. Histiocytoses. In: Kahn MF, Peltier AP, Meyer O, Piette JC (Eds) Les Maladies Systémiques. 3rd edn. Paris: Flammarion Médecine-Sciences, 1991; 891–916
2. Chu AC. Histiocytoses. In Champion RH, Burton JL, Ebling FJG (Eds) Textbook of Dermatology. 5th edn. Oxford: Blackwell Scientific Publications, 1992; 2041–2064
3. Cline MJ. Histiocytes and histiocytoses. Blood 1994; 84: 2840–2853
4. Veyssier-Belot C, Callot V. Histiocytoses. Rev Med Interne 1996; 17: 911–923
5. Van Furth R. Origin and turnover of monocytes and macrophages. Curr Top Pathol 1989; 79: 125–150
6. Jaffe R. Review of human dendritic cells. Isolation and culture from precursors. Pediatr Pathol 1993; 13: 821–837
7. Emile JF, Peuchmaur M, Fraitag S, Bodemer C, Brousse N. Immunocytochemical detection of granulocyte-macrophage stimulating factor in Langerhans cell histiocytosis. Histopathology 1993; 23: 327–332
8. Santiago-Schwarz F, Belilos E, Diamond B, Carsons SE. TNF in combination with GM-CSF enhances the differentiation of neonatal cord blood stem cells in dendritic cells and macrophages. J Leuk Biol 1992; 52: 274–281
9. Foucar K, Foucar E. The mononuclear phagocyte and immunoregulatory effector (M-PIRE) system evolving concepts. Sem Diag Pathol 1990; 7: 4–18
10. Steinman RM, Nussenzweig MC. Dendritic cells: features and functions. Immunol Rev 1980; 53: 127–147
11. Schmitt D, Dezutter-Dambuyant C, Staquet MJ, Thivolet J. La cellule de Langerhans. Méd Sci 1989; 2: 103–111
12. Stingl G, Wolf-Schreiner EC, Pichler WJ et al. Epidermal Langerhans cells bear Fc and C3 receptors. Nature 1977; 26: 245–246
13. Murphy G, Bhan AK, Sato S, Mihm MC Jr, Harrist TJ. A new immunological marker of Langerhans cells. N Engl J Med 1981; 304: 791–792
14. Rowden G, Connely EM, Winkelmann R. Cutaneous histiocytosis X. The presence of S100 protein and its use in diagnosis. Arch Dermatol 1983; 5: 145–150
15. Favara BE, Feller AC, Pauli M et al. Contemporary classification of histiocytic disorders. The WHO Committee on histiocytic/reticulum cell proliferations. Reclassification working group of the Histiocyte Society. Med Pediatr Oncol 1997; 29: 157–166
16. Woda BA, Sullivan JL. Reactive histiocytic disorders. Am J Clin Pathol 1993; 99: 459–463
17. Finan MC, Winkelmann RK. Histopathology of necrobiotic xanthogranuloma with paraproteinemia. J Cut Pathol 1987; 14: 92–99
18. Metzler G, Schlagenhauff B, Krober SM, Kaiserling E, Schaumburg-Lever GLG. Granulomatous mycosis fungoides: report of a case with some histopathologic features of granulomatous slack skin. Am J Dermatopathol 1999; 21: 156–160
19. Van Haselen CW, Toonstra J, van der Putte SJ et al. Granulomatous slack skin. Report of three patients with an updated review of the literature. Dermatology 1998; 196: 382–391
20. Favara BE. Hemophagocytic lymphohistiocytosis: a hemophagocytic syndrome. Sem Diag Pathol 1992; 9: 63–74
21. Snow JL, Su WPD. Histiocytic diseases. J Am Acad Dermatol 1995; 33: 111–116
22. McLelland J, Pritchard J, Chu AC. Current controversies. Hematol Oncol Clin N Am 1987; 1: 147–162
23. Willman CL, McClain KL. An update on clonality, cytokines, and viral etiology in Langerhans cell histiocytosis. Hematol Oncol Clin N Am 1998; 12: 407–416
24. Yu RC, Buluwela L, Chu AC. Clonal proliferation of Langerhans cells in Langerhans' cell histiocytosis. Lancet 1994; 343: 767–768
25. Willman CL, Busque L, Griffith BB. Langerhans' cell histiocytosis (histiocytosis X). A clonal proliferative disease. N Engl J Med 1994; 331: 154–160
26. The Writing Group of the Histiocyte Society. Histiocytosis syndromes in children. Lancet 1987; 1: 208–209
27. Wood GS, Haber RS. Novel histiocytoses considered in the context of histiocyte subset differentiation. Arch Dermatol 1993; 129: 210–214
28. Nezelof C, Basset F. Langerhans' cell histiocytosis research. Past, present, and future. Hematol Oncol Clin N Am 1998; 12: 385–406

29. Schmitz L, Favara BE. Nosology and pathology of Langerhans' cell histiocytosis. Hematol Oncol Clin N Am 1998; 12: 221–246

30. Emile JF, Wechsler J, Brousse N. Langerhans' cell histiocytosis: definitive diagnosis with the use of monoclonal antibody O10 on routinely paraffin-embedded samples. Am J Surg Pathol 1995; 19: 636–641

31. Neuman C, Schaumburg-Lever G, Döpfer R. Interferon gamma is a marker for histiocytosis X cells in the skin. J Invest Dermatol 1988; 91: 280–282

32. Favara BE. Langerhans' cell histiocytosis pathobiology and pathogenesis. Sem Oncol 1991; 18: 3–7

33. Groh V, Gadner H, Radaszkiewicz T. The phenotypic spectrum of histiocytosis X cells. J Invest Dermatol 1988; 90: 441–447

34. Leikin SL. Immunobiology of histiocytosis-X. Hematol Oncol Clin N Am 1987; 1: 49–61

35. Leahy MA, Brice SL, Weston WL. Langerhans' cell histiocytosis. Curr Prob Dermatol 1994; 6: 1–25

36. Longaker MA, Frieden IJ, LeBoit PE, Sherertz EF. Congenital self-healing Langerhans' cell histiocytosis: the need for long-term follow-up. J Am Acad Dermatol 1994; 31: 910–916

37. Oberman HA. Idiopathic histiocytoses: a clinicopathologic study of 40 cases and review of the literature on eosinophilic granuloma of bone, Hand–Schüller–Christian disease and Lettere–Siwe disease. Pediatrics 1961; 28: 307–327.

38. Geissmann F, Emile JF, Andry P et al. Lack of E-cathederine is associated with dissemination of Langerhans' cell histiocytosis and poor outcome. J Pathol 1997; 181: 301–304

39. Egeler RM, Neglia JP, Arico M et al. The relation of Langerhans' cell histiocytosis to acute leukemia, lymphomas, and other solid tumors. The LCH-Malignancy Study Group of the Histiocyte Society. Hematol Oncol Clin N Am 1998; 12: 369–378

40. Gianotti F, Caputo R. Histiocytic syndromes: a review. J Am Acad Dermatol 1985; 13: 383–404

41. Munn S, Chu AC. Langerhans' cell histiocytosis of the skin. Hematol Oncol Clin N Am 1998; 12: 269–286

42. Ben Azra J, Bailey A, Azumi L. Malignant histiocytosis X: a distinct entity. Cancer 1991; 68: 1050–1060

43. Zelger BWH, Sidoroff A, Orchard G, Cerio R. Non-Langerhans' cell histiocytoses. A new unifying concept. Am J Dermatopathol 1996; 18: 490–504

44. Cohen BA, Hood A. Xanthogranuloma: report on clinical and histologic findings in 64 patients. Pediatr Dermatol 1989; 6: 262–266

45. Flach DB, Winkelmann RK. Juvenile xanthogranuloma with central nervous system lesions. J Am Acad Dermatol 1986; 14: 405–411

46. Caputo R, Gianni E, Imondi D, Carminati G, Gianotti R. Papular xanthoma in children. J Am Acad Dermatol 1990; 22: 1052–1056

47. Blobstein SH, Caldwell D, Carter M. Bone lesions in xanthoma disseminatum. Arch Dermatol 1985; 121: 1313–1317

48. Battaglini J, Olsen TG. Disseminated xanthosiderohistiocytosis, a variant of xanthoma disseminatum, in a patient with a plasma cell dyscresia. J Am Acad Dermatol 1984; 11: 750–755

49. Nunnink JC, Krusinski PA, Yates JW. Multicentric reticulohistiocytosis and cancer: a case report and review of the literature. Med Pediatr Oncol 1985; 13: 273–279

50. Oliver GF, Umbert I, Winkelmann RK, Muller SA. Reticulohistiocytoma cutis: review of 15 cases and an association with systemic vasculitis in two cases. Clin Exp Dermatol 1990; 15: 1–6

51. Gianotti F, Caputo R, Ermacora E, Gianni E. Benign cephalic histiocytosis. Arch Dermatol 1986; 122: 1038–1043

52. Umbert IJ, Winkelmann RK. Eruptive histiocytoma. J Acad Dermatol 1989; 20: 958–964

53. Bork K, Hoede N. Hereditary progressive mucinous histiocytosis in women: report of three members in a family. Arch Dermatol 1988; 124: 1225–1229

54. Zina AM, Bundino S, Pippione S. Sea-blue histiocytosis with cutaneous involvement: a case report with ultrastructural findings. Dermatologica 1987; 174: 39–44

55. Berti E, Gianotti R, Alessi E. Unusual cutaneous histiocytosis expressing an indeterminate immunophenotype between Langerhans cells and dermal macrophages. Arch Dermatol 1988; 124: 1250–1253

56. Sidoroff A, Zelger B, Steiner H, Smith N. Indeterminate cell histiocytosis – a clinicopathological entity with features of both X- and non-X histiocytosis. Br J Dermatol 1996; 134: 525–532

57. Romani N, Lenz A, Glassel H et al. Cultured human Langerhans cells resemble lymphoid dendritic cells in phenotype and function. J Invest Dermatol 1989; 93: 600–609

58. Teunissen MBM, Wormmeester J, Krieg SR et al. Human epidermal Langerhans cells undergo profound morphologic and phenotypical changes during in vitro culture. J Invest Dermatol 1990; 94: 166–173

59. Murphy GF, Messadi D, Fonferko E, Hancock WW. Phenotypic transformation of macrophages to Langerhans cells in the skin. Am J Pathol 1986; 123: 401–406

60. Chu P, LeBoit PE. Histologic features of cutaneous sinus histiocytosis (Rosai–Dorfman disease): study of cases both with and without systemic involvement. J Cut Pathol 1992; 19: 201–206

61. Perrin C, Michiels JF, Lacour JP, Chagnon A, Fuzibet JG. Sinus histiocytosis clinically limited to the skin. J Cut Pathol 1993; 20: 368–374

62. Rozenberg I, Wechsler J, Koenig F et al. Maladie d'Erdheim–Chester. Forme multiviscérale révélée par une exophtalmie. Rev Med Interne 1986; 7: 311–317

63. Pertuiset E, Laredo JD, Liote D et al. Erdheim–Chester disease: report of a case. Review of the literature and discussion of relationships with Langerhans' cell histiocytosis. Rev Rhum, Edition Française 1993; 60: 601–609

64. Brower AC, Worsham GF, Dudley AH. Erdheim–Chester disease: a distinct lipoidosis or part of the spectrum of histiocytosis? Radiology 1984; 151: 35–38

65. Veyssier-Belot C, Cacoub P, Caparros-Lefebvre D et al. Erdheim–Chester disease. Clinical and radiologic characteristics of 59 cases. Medicine 1996; 75: 157–169

66. Wilson MS, Weiss LM, Gatter KC. Malignant histiocytosis: a reassessment of cases previously reported in 1975 based on paraffin section immunophenotyping studies. Cancer 1990; 66: 530–536

67. Kamel OW, Gocke CD, Kell DL, Cleary ML, Warnke RA. True histiocytic lymphoma: a study of 12 cases based on current definition. Leuk Lymph 1995; 18: 81–86

68. Ruco LP, Pulford KA, Mason DY et al. Expression of macrophage-associated antigens in tissues involved by Langerhans' cell histiocytosis (histiocytosis X). Am J Clin Pathol 1989; 92: 273–279

4

Sentinel lymph node pathology

Alistair J. Cochran

INTRODUCTION

This chapter draws on our considerable experience of the techniques of lymphatic mapping and sentinel node dissection and provides recommendations similar to those contained in previous articles.[1,2] Management of primary melanoma is generally agreed to be excision of the primary tumour with a margin of surrounding normal skin. In contrast, there is little consensus as to whether and when the regional lymph nodes should be excised in patients with high-risk (deep, thick) primary melanomas. Some consider that ipsilateral regional nodes should be excised when the primary is removed; i.e. *elective or prophylactic lymphadenectomy*.[3-6] Arguments in favour of this approach include the substantially better survival of patients with melanoma confined to the primary site, in comparison with patients with tumour in the regional nodes and the observation that 20–30% of patients with clinically uninvolved nodes have melanoma in the excised nodes, on examination by histology and immunohistology.[7] A major argument against this approach is that, if all individuals with high-risk melanoma are subjected to elective lymphadenectomy, 70–80% will receive an unnecessary surgical operation that carries significant morbidity and a small possibility of operation-associated death. Others[8-12] consider that lymphadenectomy should be reserved for patients who develop clinically evident tumour in the nodes (*therapeutic lymphadenectomy*). This spares many patients an unnecessary operation, but delays definitive therapy for the minority of patients who may benefit from early lymphadenectomy and deprives these individuals of their best chance of cure.

We have long considered that a proportion of patients with high-risk primary melanoma would benefit from early and elective nodal dissection. These patients are likely to have limited nodal metastases and absent or minimal systemic

Alistair J. Cochran MD FRCP(glasg), FRCPath, Professor of Pathology and Surgery, 13–145 CHS, Department of Pathology and Laboratory Medicine, UCLA School of Medicine, 10833 Le Conte Avenue, Los Angeles, California 90095–1732, USA

spread. Until recently we could not identify these individuals, and this dictated lymphadenectomy for all patients with high-risk melanoma, imposing an unnecessary operation on many.

We have now developed the techniques necessary for identifying those individuals who are likely to benefit from lymphadenectomy. We needed to be able to identify very small numbers of tumour cells in tissues, including lymph nodes. This became possible after our development of S-100 protein[13] as a marker for melanocytic tumours[14–18] and the appearance of antibodies to melanoma-associated epitopes, such as HMB-45,[19] NKI/C3[20] and Melan-A.[21,22] We have demonstrated that conventional histology underestimates by 14% the number of patients with primary melanoma localized to the site of origin by clinical assessment who, in fact, have early metastatic melanoma in the regional nodes.[7] Conventional histology also underestimates by 30% tumour-positivity in ostensibly tumour-free nodes of patients with node spread melanoma.[23] In patients with nodal tumour identifiable only by immunohistology, the number of nodes containing occult tumour cells was small (usually only one or two) and the number of tumour cells present in an individual node was also small. Consideration of the anatomical site of nodes containing occult micrometastases required their careful orientation relative to the primary tumour.[24,25] The nodes that contained occult tumour were found to be located close to the primary melanoma.

To develop a better approach to the treatment of high-risk primary melanoma, we also needed to be able to identify in vivo, the nodes most likely to contain tumour. We have had a long-standing interest in lymphoscintigraphy (with technetium-labelled albumin or dextran), which accurately identifies the node group to which lymph drains from a particular anatomical site.[26] Identification of the individual nodes within a node group that are most likely to contain tumour is more difficult. We developed an animal model in which a marker dye injected intradermally passed reliably from comparable areas of skin to a predictable regional lymph node.[27] Application of this approach to patients with melanoma showed that it was possible to identify blue coloured afferent lymphatics and one or more 'sentinel' lymph nodes in many patients (lymphatic mapping). We consider the sentinel node to be the first lymph node on the direct lymphatic pathway from the site of the primary melanoma. The anatomical position of the sentinel node is thus unique to the individual. The use of a 'sentinel node' as a means of directing nodal surgery for penile carcinoma was previously reported by Cabanas (1977).[28] We developed the techniques of lymphatic mapping and selective lymph node dissection for melanoma[29] by combining the findings of these various studies.

The sentinel node is identified by lymphatic mapping using a dye and a radioactive marker. The nodal tissues are closely evaluated by histology and immunohistochemistry for metastatic melanoma. If the sentinel node contains tumour, a complete lymphadenectomy is undertaken. In the absence of melanoma further surgery is not performed and the patient is regularly observed.

This technique has generated considerable enthusiasm among surgical oncologists and there are now many reports of its successful application.[30–35] A prospective trial of this approach for melanoma has been funded by the US National Cancer Institute, comparing selective lymph node dissection with a 'watch and wait' approach after wide excision.

Surgical pathologists are increasingly requested to examine tissues removed during this type of procedure. To assist those asked to evaluate such tissues, we describe our experience of the pathological aspects of selective lymph node dissection and provide recommendations based on our experience and on the published literature.

MATERIAL AND METHODS

The recommendations in this chapter are based on our experience with 1119 sentinel lymph nodes from 446 patients entered into an ongoing National Cancer Institute multicentre trial of sentinel lymph node dissection directed by the John Wayne Cancer Institute, Santa Monica, California.

For each patient we determined the following: (i) the number of sentinel lymph nodes provided; (ii) the number of sentinel lymph nodes identified as containing tumour on examination of haematoxylin and eosin (H&E) stained slides; (iii) the number of sentinel lymph nodes identified as containing tumour in sections stained by immunoperoxidase techniques using antibodies to S-100 protein and HMB-45. Where we have information on the lymph nodes removed during completion lymph node dissections (all pretrial and trial patients with tumour-containing sentinel lymph nodes) we have recorded the number of non-sentinel lymph nodes that contained tumour.

IS THE NODE TRULY SENTINEL?

Since the sentinel node is the most likely site of early metastases it is of great importance that the node examined is truly the sentinel node. Determination that a node is sentinel at present depends on information from the surgeon who will rely on the localization provided by pre-operative lymphoscintigraphy,[26,28] blue colouration of afferent lymphatics and associated lymph node(s),[29] and enhanced radioactivity of the lymph node detected by a hand-held Geiger counter.[36] The pathologist should examine the submitted lymph nodes closely for the presence of the blue colouration that will confirm them as sentinel. In some instances, the whole lymph node may not be blue coloured, colour being localized to one half of the node or more limited segments. Although sentinel nodes are preferentially the site of early metastases, tumour status cannot reliably be used to confirm sentinel node status since not all sentinel nodes contain tumour and some non-sentinel nodes contain tumour (but always in association with a tumour-positive sentinel node). We are currently developing approaches that will allow pathologists to confirm, independently, whether a node is truly sentinel.

FROZEN SECTIONS

We developed the sentinel lymph node technique by using intraoperative interpretation of frozen sections. Assessment of tumour status was based on the evaluation of sections stained by H&E and sections stained by S-100 protein and HMB-45, using a rapid immunoperoxidase technique. If the sentinel node was judged to be positive, a complete lymph node dissection was undertaken. As the technique has evolved we have moved away from using frozen sections, believing that the 'facing up' required to obtain a full face frozen section preparation is wasteful of the tissue in which there is the greatest likelihood that occult tumour cells will be present.[7] Additionally, the interpretation of H&E stained frozen sections and sections stained using the rapid immunohistology approach is always more difficult and thus more error-prone than the interpretation of well-fixed 'permanent' material. We strongly recommend that interpretation of sentinel nodes is based on well-fixed full-face sections cut as close to the mid-line of the lymph node as possible.

There is a theoretical argument to be made that each sentinel lymph node should be serially sectioned to extinction, but such an approach would be impossibly expensive and is clearly impractical. Any practical recommendation must thus be a compromise between the ideal and the possible. Our present recommendation is that the lymph node is cut into two exactly equal halves through the longest circumference of the node (Fig. 4.1). These two portions of the lymph node are placed cut face down in cassettes and fixed for at least 24 hours. The technician is instructed to minimize 'facing-up'. As soon as a full-faced section can be obtained, 10 serial sections are removed. Sections 1, 3, 5 and 10 × 3 are stained by H&E, section 2 by S-100 protein, and section 4 by HMB-45. Sections 6 and 7 are used as negative controls for the immunoperoxidase studies and

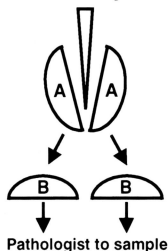

Pathologist to sample

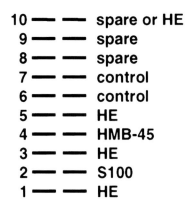

10	spare or HE
9	spare
8	spare
7	control
6	control
5	HE
4	HMB-45
3	HE
2	S100
1	HE

Fig. 4.1 The sentinel node (A) is cut into two exactly equal halves through its longest circumference. The two halves of the node (B) are placed cut face down and ten serial 'full face' sections are cut from each. (Technicians are requested to minimize tissue removed during the 'facing up' process.) Sections 1, 3, 5 and 10 are stained by H&E. Section 2 is stained with an antibody to S-100 protein and section 4 with the antibody HMB-45 (or Melan-A). Sections 6 and 7 are used as controls and sections 8 and 9 are spares for any required repeats of unsatisfactory sections.

sections 8 and 9 are available to repeat any of the studies that are technically unsatisfactory or for additional immunohistochemistry. If suspicious or anomalous appearances are seen within the first 10 sections, additional groups of 10 sections can be examined.

THE USE OF IMMUNOHISTOCHEMISTRY

All sentinel lymph nodes must be examined by immunohistology using antibodies to S-100 protein and HMB-45 or MART-1 (Melan-A), unless the node contains overt tumour on gross inspection or review of H&E stained slides. Immunohistology will always increase the frequency of sentinel lymph nodes found to contain tumour. The proportion of sentinel nodes that requires immunohistology to identify occult tumour sharply decreases as pathologists gain experience in evaluating sentinel nodes. This is the pathologists' equivalent of the surgeons' 'learning curve'.[29]

IMMUNOHISTOLOGY WITH S-100 PROTEIN

S-100 protein is a highly robust marker for melanoma cells, staining virtually 100% of melanomas.[16,18] We look for epithelioid, oval or spindle-shaped cells (usually located in the subcapsular sinus), which show S-100 protein positivity in both the cytoplasm and the nucleus (Fig. 4.2A–C). Other cells within the lymph nodes contain S-100 protein. The dendritic leukocytes of the paracortex are the most prominent of these confounding cells. Identification of these cells is not difficult in reactive paracortices where they are polydendritic (Fig. 4.2D). Difficulty may be encountered in inactive lymph nodes where the dendritic leukocytes show either no or minimal dendrite formation (Fig. 4.2E). S-100 protein positivity may also be found in capsular nevi (Fig. 4.2F–H)[37] and in the Schwann cells of node-associated nerves (Fig. 4.2I).[38]

IMMUNOHISTOLOGY WITH HMB-45

HMB-45 is a more specific marker for melanoma cells, but the cells of between 10 and 15% of melanomas (especially metastatic melanoma) do not express this epitope. In contrast to S-100 protein, HMB-45 positive epitopes are confined to the cytoplasm. Antibodies to HMB-45 have the distinct advantage that they do not stain dendritic leukocytes and either do not stain capsular nevocytes or stain them at relatively low intensity. The antibody MART-1 (Melan-A) may be used in a similar role to that of HMB-45, but suffers from the same defect in that a proportion of melanomas do not stain positively with this reagent. We have utilized HMB-45 as our second antibody throughout the development of this technique and have found no compelling reason to change to MART-1.

One potential source of error with HMB-45 is that in lymph nodes with trabecular calcification (mainly in the groin or iliac area) extracellular HMB-45 reactivity may be identified.

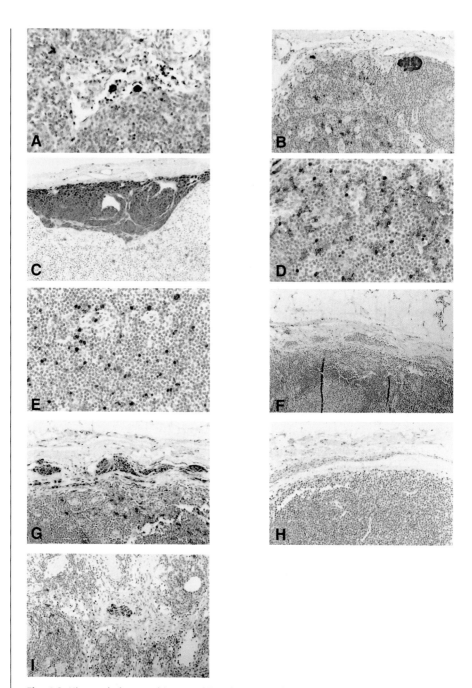

Fig. 4.2 Histopathology and immunohistochemistry of the sentinel node. **(A)** Single 'occult' metastatic melanoma cells (S-100 protein/haematoxylin). **(B)** A 'microcolony' of metastatic melanoma in the subcapsular sinus (S-100 protein/haematoxylin). **(C)** A larger colony of metastatic melanoma in a sentinel node (S-100 protein/haematoxylin). **(D)** Polydendritic dendritic leukocytes in a reactive paracortical area (S-100 protein/ haematoxylin). **(E)** Non-dendritic and parvi-dendritic dendritic leukocytes in a weakly reactive paracortical area (S-100 protein/haematoxylin). **(F)** Capsular nevus in a sentinel node (H&E). **(G)** Capsular nevus in a sentinel node (S-100 protein/haematoxylin). **(H)** Capsular nevus in a sentinel node (HMB-45/haematoxylin). **(I)** Nerve within a lymph node (S-100 protein/haematoxylin).

HANDLING OF SENTINEL NODES IDENTIFIED BY RADIOISOTOPIC LABELLING

The isotope used is generally technetium 99, which has short penetration and a short half-life. The risk to operating room personnel and pathology staff and faculty members from this radiation source is considered slight, but after bisection of the nodes it is prudent to place them in a safe place in formalin for 24 hours after surgical excision. We leave them in the care of our nuclear medicine colleagues.

RESULTS

STUDIES OF SENTINEL LYMPH NODES PRIOR TO THE MULTICENTRE TRIAL

In these early studies sentinel lymph node identification was followed by complete lymph node dissection regardless of the tumour status of the sentinel node. We evaluated 259 sentinel lymph nodes from 223 patients, an average of 1.2 sentinel lymph nodes per individual. Tumour was identified in 47 out of these 259 sentinel lymph nodes (18%). Tumour cells were identified by H&E alone in 83.2% of patients with positive sentinel nodes and in the remaining 16.7% by immunohistology alone. The tumour cells occurred as single cells (Fig. 4.2A), small clumps of tumour cells (Fig. 4.2B) and as larger colonies (Fig. 4.2C). We have found tumour in a non-sentinel node in the absence of tumour in the sentinel node in only two patients who were encountered very early in our experience with the technique. Since this situation has not been encountered subsequently, it is likely that in these two patients the true sentinel lymph node was not correctly identified.

As noted above, all patients in the pre-trial group, regardless of the tumour status of their sentinel lymph node, received a completion lymph node dissection. We identified tumour–containing non-sentinel nodes in 33% of patients with positive sentinel nodes. We usually saw tumour in a single non-sentinel node, less often in two or three. The amount of tumour in these non-sentinel nodes was generally small and was distributed as single cells or small microcolonies, almost always in the subcapsular sinus.

THE MULTICENTRE SELECTIVE LYMPH NODE TRIAL

These 446 patients represent the first series of patients entered into the trial, which will eventually comprise 1600 patients. In this group, 860 sentinel lymph nodes were removed from 512 lymph node basins, and 99 sentinel nodes contained tumour (19% positive when analysed by lymph node basin). Tumour was identified in 85 nodes by H&E histology (86%) and in the remaining 14 nodes by immunohistology (14%).

PITFALLS IN INTERPRETING SENTINEL LYMPH NODES

S-100 PROTEIN STAINING

The major problem here is the interpretation of S-100 positive dendritic leukocytes in the paracortex or sinuses. Dendritic leukocyte identification (Fig. 4.2D) may be especially difficult if the dendritic leukocytes are non-dendritic, as is often the case in immune suppressed inactive sentinel nodes (Fig. 4.2E). With good quality immunohistochemical preparations, sinus macrophages do not stain for S-100 protein. However, if there is background staining, these cells may present interpretative difficulties. Capsular nevocytes (Fig. 4.2F) occur in more than 20% of patients undergoing sentinel lymph node dissection and are made more visible by the use of immunohistochemistry (Fig. 4.2G). Capsular nevocytes are confined to the capsule and trabeculae of the lymph node. They are smaller and more cohesive than melanoma cells (with the possible exception of nevocytoid melanoma) and, while strongly S-100 protein positive, express HMB-45 at a relatively weak level or not at all (Fig. 4.2H). Nevocytes often cluster around capsular vessels. The presence of neural tissue within the lymph node may occasionally cause interpretative difficulty (Fig. 4.2I). If the nerve has associated Schwann cells, these may stain relatively strongly with S-100 protein and if the nerve is cut transversely an appearance suggestive of a cluster of S-100 protein positive melanoma cells may result.

HMB-45 STAINING

The main problem with this reagent is the fact that in a proportion of melanomas (10–15%) the tumour cells are unreactive with HMB-45. In hyalinized and calcified connective tissue within lymph nodes, especially lymph nodes from the groin and internal iliac areas, extracellular HMB-45 positivity may be seen and care is necessary to avoid overcalling this appearance.

DISCUSSION

Sentinel lymph node technology has become very widely adopted in the relatively few years since we first described the application of this technique to melanoma.[29] There is as yet no evidence that this approach is therapeutic. The technique certainly represents a considerable improvement in our ability to evaluate the tumour status of the regional lymph nodes for prognostication and may be useful in selecting patients for adjuvant therapy. Information as to the therapeutic relevance of the approach must await the outcome of the multicentre trial (ca 2003). While the concept of the approach is appealing and the techniques seem simple from the surgical, pathological and nuclear medicine standpoints, there are clearly pitfalls. The technique is also being used in a variety of other cancers including breast cancer, colon cancer and vulvar carcinoma. It was previously applied to penile carcinoma.[28] While the broad lessons learned from our extensive experience with melanoma are probably applicable to other tumour systems, we urge caution and care in developing the techniques for each individual cancer system.

One proof of the effectiveness of the approach will be the frequency at which patients develop metastases in the ipsilateral regional nodes after removal of a reportedly negative lymph node. In our experience, this is infrequent. We have six patients in whom ipsilateral regional failure occurred despite an allegedly negative sentinel node. Detailed re-examination of the pathological material and clinical records of these individuals indicated that in three patients a tumour-positive sentinel lymph node had initially been incorrectly interpreted as negative. In one case a few single tumour cells were missed. In two cases, tumour was not visible on the original H&E preparation and in neither case was immunohisto-chemistry performed. It is likely that if immunoperoxidase preparations had been examined a correct interpretation would have been made in each of these patients. In the remaining three patients, despite extensive sampling of the 'sentinel' lymph node by H&E staining and immunohistochemistry, no evidence of tumour was identified. It is likely that the surgeons did not correctly identify the sentinel nodes in these patients.

It is, therefore, essential to identify the sentinel lymph node with high accuracy. While, for the moment, this remains primarily the responsibility of the surgeon, the process has been rendered more accurate by a three-step sequence. The patient is subjected to a lymphoscintigraphy prior to operation, in which an early reading is made immediately after introduction of the isotope. This permits the identification of the sentinel node, the site of which can be identified by a tattoo on the skin, providing guidance to the surgeon in making the initial incision. Operating surgeons, in addition to injecting blue dye in the area of the primary melanoma often include technetium-labelled albumin, which generates enhanced radioactivity in the sentinel node. Techniques are being developed to allow pathologists to accurately confirm the sentinel status of a submitted lymph node.

Accurate determination of the tumour status of the sentinel lymph node is also essential. This depends on careful sampling of the node and the routine use and accurate interpretation of immunohistochemical preparations. The technique that we recommend (Fig. 4.1) has served us well and is probably sufficient for the great majority of patients. In specific subsets of patients with unusually deep or thick melanoma, additional sampling may be necessary. Studies are in progress to evaluate that possibility.

There is much interest in the possibility that in evaluating nodes for the presence of tumour, molecular biological techniques may provide information that is additional to that provided by conventional pathology and immunohistochemistry. In considering these claims, it is necessary to recognize that conventional pathology and immunohistology identify slightly less than 20% of sentinel nodes as containing tumour and that in patients treated by wide local excision alone, the regional failure rate is at a similar frequency. Molecular biologists claim that by using Reverse Transcriptase Polymerase Chain Reaction (RTPCR) technology they can identify signals for mRNA species (which may be associated with metastatic melanoma cells) in a proportion of lymph nodes where evaluation of H&E and immunohistochemistry preparations has not demonstrated tumour. This work was initially undertaken using primers for m-tyrosinase and it is widely accepted that cells other than metastatic melanoma cells contain mRNA for tyrosinase, including capsular nevocytes and Schwann cells in node-associated nerves. Thus the demonstration of a signal for tyrosinase mRNA cannot be interpreted as certainly indicating the presence of metastatic melanoma. Studies in progress, in which multiple primers (for example to mRNA for MUC18 or MART-1) are used, represent a scientifically more interesting approach. The need to evaluate the role and significance of molecular biology in the analysis of sentinel nodes is clear. Pathologists should, however, be careful to avoid providing sentinel lymph node tissue for scientific study in a manner that may compromise diagnosis. It is inappropriate arbitrarily to provide portions of a sentinel lymph node for research. We prefer to provide sections cut from the lymph node in a serial fashion and interspersed with sections stained by H&E and those used for immunohistology. This approach has the additional advantage that it facilitates interpretation of the RTPCR results, by allowing close morphological comparison.

Sentinel lymph node technology has much to offer melanoma patients in terms of staging and may have a therapeutic role. The technology will be investigated and exploited in many different tumour systems. Pathologists have a key role in evaluating the effectiveness of the approach. Careful attention to sampling and interpretation of the sentinel nodes is mandatory.

KEY POINTS

1. Patients with high-risk (thick, deeply invasive) primary melanoma have, in the past, been managed by wide local excision and elective node dissection or wide local excision alone, with lymphadenectomy only when the regional nodes develop metastases that are clinically detectable.
2. We have recently developed an alternative surgical approach, selective lymph node dissection.
3. Here, a marker dye (isosulphan blue) usually combined with a radioactive marker (technetium–labelled albumin), is injected intradermally in the tissues around the primary melanoma. The afferent lymphatics are tracked to the first lymph node(s) in the ipsilateral regional lymph node area. The surgeon excises the blue-coloured and maximally radioactive 'sentinel node(s)' and the pathologist evaluates these for metastatic tumour. If the sentinel nodes are tumour free, further nodal dissection is not undertaken; if tumour is present, a formal complete dissection of the nodal basin is performed.
4. We have examined 1119 sentinel lymph nodes from 669 patients treated by selective lymph node dissection as part of a trial of the technique. We identified melanoma cells in lymphadenectomy specimens from 126 patients (17.8%). Furthermore, 67% of specimens contained a single positive node, 25% had two positive nodes and the remaining 12% had three. We encountered melanoma cells dispersed singly or arranged in small groups, almost always in the peripheral sinus. A proportion of cases (~4%) required immunohistochemistry to identify truly minute numbers of tumour cells.
5. With experience pathologists can identify tumour in an increasing proportion of lymph nodes in H&E preparations.
6. Occult nodal tumour cells are more frequent in patients with primary tumours of deeper Clark level and greater Breslow thickness.
7. Tumour cells have to be discriminated from capsular nevus cells, interdigitating dendritic leukocytes, macrophages and intranodal neural tissues.

8. With experience and the use of immunohistochemistry the detection of small numbers of melanoma cells in sentinel nodes is a comparatively straightforward exercise.
9. Extensive research is currently underway using sentinel lymph node technology in a variety of other cancers.
10. Techniques are being developed to aid pathologists in accurately confirming sentinel status of a lymph node and in accurately determining tumour status.
11. Research is also needed to evaluate the role and significance of molecular biological techniques in the analysis of sentinel nodes.

REFERENCES

1. Cochran AJ, Morton DL, Wen D-R. The surgical pathology of dye-directed selective lymph node dissection. In Nieweg OE, Essner R, Reintgen DS (Eds) Lymphatic Mapping. New York: Marcel Dekker 2000; 125–140
2. Cochran AJ. Surgical pathology remains pivotal in the evaluation of 'sentinel' lymph nodes. Am J Surg Pathol 2000; 23: 1169–1172
3. Goldsmith HS, Shah JP, Kim DH. Prognostic significance of lymph node dissection in the treatment of malignant melanoma. Cancer 1970; 26: 606–609
4. Day CL, Mihm MC, Lew RA et al. Prognostic factors for patients with clinical Stage I melanoma of intermediate thickness (1.5–3.99 mm). Ann Surg 1982; 195: 35–43
5. Balch CM. The role of elective lymph node dissection in melanoma: rationale, results and controversies. J Clin Oncol 1988; 6: 163–172
6. Balch CM, Soong S-J, Bartolucci AA et al. Efficacy of an elective regional lymph node dissection of 1 to 4 mm thick melanomas for patients 60 years of age and younger. Ann Surg 1996; 224: 255–266
7. Cochran AJ, Wen D-R, Morton DL. Occult tumor cells in the lymph nodes of patients with pathological stage I malignant melanoma: an immunohistological study. Am J Surg Pathol 1988; 12: 612–618
8 Veronesi U, Adamus J, Bandiera DC et al. Inefficacy of immediate node dissection in stage I melanoma of the limbs. N Engl J Med 1977; 297: 627–630
9. Veronesi U, Adamus J, Bandiera DC et al. Delayed regional lymph node dissection in stage I melanoma of the skin of the lower extremities. Cancer 1982; 49: 2420–2430
10. Sim FH, Taylor WF, Ivins JC et al. A prospective, randomized study of the efficacy of routine elective lymphadenectomy in the management of melanoma. Cancer 1978; 41: 948–956
11. Cady B. 'Prophylactic' lymph node dissection on melanoma: does it help? J Clin Oncol 1988; 6: 2–4
12. Coats AS, Ingvar CI, Peterson-Schaefer K et al. Elective lymph node dissection in patients with primary melanoma of the trunk and limbs treated at the Sydney Melanoma Unit from 1960 to 1991. J. Amer Coll Surg 1995; 180: 402–409
13. Moore BW. Chemistry and biology of two proteins, S-100 and 14–3–2, specific to the nervous system. Biochem Biophys Res Commun 1965; 19: 739–744
14. Gaynor R, Irie R, Morton DL, Herschman HR. S-100 protein in cultured human malignant melanomas. Nature 1980; 286: 400–401
15. Gaynor R, Herschman HR, Irie R et al. S-100 protein: a marker for human malignant melanomas? Lancet 1981; 1: 869–871
16. Cochran AJ, Wen D-R, Herschman HR, Gaynor RB. Detection of S-100 protein as an aid to the identification of melanocytic tumors. Int J Cancer 1982; 30: 295–297
17. Cochran AJ, Holland G, Wen D-R et al. Detection of S-100 protein in the diagnosis of primary and metastatic intraocular tumors. Invest Ophthalmol Vis Sci 1983; 24: 1153–1155
18. Wen D-R, Gaynor RB, Cochran AJ. S-100 protein: a marker for melanocytic tumors. Ann N Y Acad Sci 1983; 420: 261–266

19. Gown AM, Vogel AM, Heak D, Gough D, McNutt MA. Monoclonal antibodies specific for melanocyte tumors distinguished subpopulations of melanocytes. Am J Pathol 1986; 123: 195–203

20. Hagen EC, Vennegoor C, Schlingemann RO, Van der Velde ER, Ruiter DJ. Correlation of histopathological characteristics with staining patterns in human malignant melanoma assessed by (monoclonal) antibodies reactive on paraffin sections. Histopathology 1986; 10: 689–700

21. Chen Y-T, Stockert E, Jungblith A et al. Serological analysis of Melan-A (MART-1), a melanocyte-specific protein homogenously expressed in human melanomas. Proc Natl Acad Sci USA 1996; 93: 5915–5919

22. Fetsch PA, Cromier J, Hijazi YM. Immunocytochemical detections of MART-1 in fresh and paraffin embedded malignant melanomas. J Immunother 1997; 20: 60–64

23. Cochran AJ, Wen D-R, Herschman HR. Occult melanoma in lymph nodes detected by antiserum to S-100 protein. Int J Cancer 1984; 34: 159–163

24. Cochran AJ, Pihl E, Wen D-R, Hoon DSB, Korn EL. Zoned immune suppression of lymph nodes draining malignant melanoma: histologic and immunohistologic studies. J Natl Cancer Inst 1987; 78: 399–405

25. Hoon DSB, Korn EL, Cochran AJ. Variations in functional immunocompetence of human tumor-draining lymph nodes. Cancer Res 1987; 47: 1740–1744

26. Robinson DS, Sample WF, Fee JH et al. Regional lymphatic drainage in primary malignant melanoma of the trunk determined by colloidal gold scanning. Surg Forum 1977; 28: 147–148

27. Wong JH, Cagle LA, Morton DL. Lymphatic drainage of skin to a sentinel lymph node in a feline model. Ann Surg 1991; 214: 637–641

28. Cabanas RM. An approach to the treatment of penile carcinoma. Cancer 1977; 39: 456–466

29. Morton DL, Wen D-R, Wong JH et al. Technical details of intraoperative lymphatic mapping for early stage melanoma. Arch Surg 1992; 127: 392–399

30. Reintgen D. More rational and conservative surgical strategies for malignant melanoma using lymphatic mapping and sentinel node biopsy techniques. Curr Opin Oncol 1996; 8: 152–158

31. Leong SP, Steinmetz I, Habib FA et al. Optimal selective sentinel lymph node dissection in primary malignant melanoma. Arch Surg 1997; 132: 666–672

32. Lingam MK, Mackie RM, McKay AJ. Intraoperative identification of sentinel lymph node in patients with malignant melanoma. Br J Cancer 1997; 75: 1505–1508

33. Nieweg OE, Kapteijn BA, Thompson JF, Kroon BB. Lymphatic mapping and selective lymphadenectomy for melanoma: not yet standard therapy. Eur J Surg Oncol 1997; 23: 397–398

34. Ross MI. Lymphatic mapping and sentinel node biopsy for early stage melanoma: how we do it at the M.D. Anderson Cancer Center. J Surg Oncol 1997; 66: 273–276

35. Bostick P, Essner R, Sarantou T et al. Intraoperative lymphatic mapping for early-stage melanoma of the head and neck. Am J Surg 1997; 174: 536–539

36. Nathanson SD, Anaya P, Karvelis KC, Eck L, Havstad S. Sentinel lymph node uptake of two different technetium-labeled radiocolloids. Ann Surg Oncol 1996; 4: 104–110

37. Carson KF, Wen D-R, Li P-X et al. Nodal nevi and cutaneous melanomas. Am J Surg Pathol 1996; 20: 834–840

38. Cochran AJ, Bailly C, Paul E, Remotti F. Melanocytic Tumors: A Guide to Diagnosis. Philadelphia and New York: Lippincott-Raven, 1997

5

The clinical and molecular pathology of Barrett's oesophagus

L.R. Biddlestone T.A. Bailey C.E. Whittles N.A. Shepherd

INTRODUCTION

Barrett's oesophagus has aroused increasing interest over recent years, largely because of its recognition as a risk factor for the development of oesophageal adenocarcinoma. The past few decades have seen a dramatic increase in the incidence of adenocarcinoma of the oesophagus and the gastric cardia. Currently this tumour has a poor prognosis when presenting symptomatically. Hence surveillance of Barrett's oesophagus patients, with the aim of early detection of glandular neoplasia, has been advocated. Advances in the understanding of the molecular mechanisms involved in the metaplasia–dysplasia–adenocarcinoma sequence may result in the development of markers of early stages of carcinogenesis and this, in combination with surveillance, may allow the identification of patients at risk and earlier intervention. There is also interest in the use of novel medical therapies and local ablation techniques to destroy the metaplastic columnar mucosa in the oesophagus in the hope of reducing their cancer risk. Thus the practising histopathologist has an ever-increasing role in the histological corroboration of the endoscopic diagnosis of columnar lined oesophagus (CLO), in the identification of neoplastic change and in the monitoring of response to these newer treatment modalities.

Leigh R. Biddlestone MBChB MRCPath, Consultant Histopathologist and Cytopathologist, Royal United Hospital, Bath, UK

Tracey A. Bailey BSc (Hons) PhD, Post-doctoral Scientist, Department of Pathology, Institute of Ophthalmology, University College London, Bath Street, London, EC1V 9EL, UK

Cheryl E. Whittles PhD former PhD student, Biotechnology Centre and The Gloucestershire Royal and Cranfield University Institute of Medical Sciences, Cranfield University, UK

Neil A. Shepherd MB BS FRCPath, Consultant Histopathologist, Department of Histopathology, Gloucestershire Royal Hospital, Great Western Road, Gloucester, GL1 3NN, UK and Visiting Professor in Histopathology, Cranfield University, UK

EPIDEMIOLOGY

The prevalence of traditional Barrett's oesophagus, defined as greater than 3 cm of CLO, in the general population has been estimated at 376/100 000 from an autopsy study.[1] This is more than 17 times the clinically diagnosed prevalence, emphasizing the fact that the great majority of CLO patients remain undetected. Around 1% of patients undergoing upper gastrointestinal (GI) endoscopy for any reason have CLO and 3–7% of those presenting with reflux symptoms will have biopsy-proven CLO. The prevalence increases with age to about 1% at age 60 years. The last two decades have seen a sharp rise in the incidence of CLO, especially in the UK: whilst this can partly be related to increased endoscopic activity and recognition, there is little doubt that there has been true and exponential increase in CLO incidence.[2]

Much of the increased interest in CLO has stemmed from the rapidly rising incidence of oesophageal adenocarcinoma (Fig. 5.1). Blot et al[3] reported a three-fold increase in incidence comparing 1988–1990 with 1976–1978 and a population–based study showed a five to sixfold increase in both oesophageal and gastric cardiac adenocarcinoma between 1935–1971 and 1974–1989.[4] The increased risk of adenocarcinoma of the oesophagus in patients with CLO is variously estimated at between a 30 and 125-fold increase compared with an age-matched population without CLO.[1] The incidence of adenocarcinoma in CLO is estimated at between 1 in 100 and 1 in 180 patient-years.[1,5–8] The dramatic, indeed epidemic, increase in oesophageal adenocarcinoma, has resulted in oesophageal cancer, as a whole, becoming the fifth commonest cancer killer in males in the UK this decade.

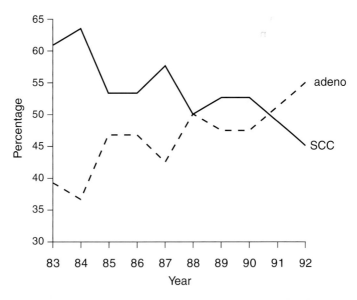

Fig. 5.1 The comparison of the incidence of squamous cell carcinoma (SCC) and adenocarcinoma (adeno) of the oesophagus in one decade in the South West Region, UK. The incidence of squamous cell carcinoma has remained relatively static: this emphasizes the exponential increase in oesophageal adenocarcinoma in 10 years. Data from the South West Cancer Registry, 1983–1992.

HISTORICAL PERSPECTIVES AND DEFINITIONS

In 1950 Mr Norman Barrett, a St Thomas' Hospital (London) surgeon, described 'chronic peptic ulcer of the oesophagus',[9] although a similar condition had been described as early as 1839. He suggested that these peptic ulcers arising in gastric-type columnar mucosa were actually cases of congenitally short oesophagus with ulceration occurring in the proximal stomach which had been displaced into the thorax. Barrett's report included no mention of intestinal metaplasia: Bosher & Taylor[10] and Morson & Belcher[11] are credited with the first descriptions of goblet cells in the columnar lined oesophagus, the latter in a patient with oesophageal adenocarcinoma.[12] Subsequently it was proposed that the columnar lined mediastinal structure was oesophagus rather than stomach and, in 1957, Barrett conceded that this was indeed the case and proposed the term 'lower oesophagus lined by columnar epithelium'.[12,13] Increasing evidence became available that CLO was an acquired condition, rather than congenital, and was primarily related to the reflux of gastric, and later gastroduodenal, contents into the oesophagus.

The lack of a universally accepted definition of Barrett's oesophagus has resulted in confusion and difficulties in comparing different studies of this condition. The various definitions of Barrett's oesophagus have included both endoscopic and histological criteria. In most cases of traditional/classical CLO, the diagnosis is usually very obvious at endoscopy (Fig. 5.2) and histological

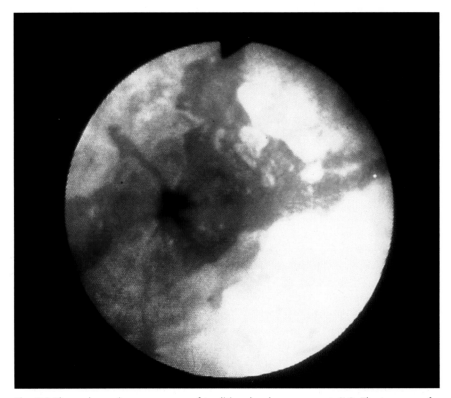

Fig. 5.2 The endoscopic appearances of traditional or long segment CLO. The tongues of salmon pink mucosa of the CLO contrast with the white squamous mucosa of the oesophagus. Histology would merely be corroborative to the endoscopic diagnosis of CLO.

assessment is merely a corroborative exercise. In earlier studies, biopsies taken from endoscopically identified CLO showed a range of histological appearances including atrophic gastric fundic mucosa, cardiac mucosa and glandular mucosa with goblet cells indicating intestinal metaplasia. However if biopsies are taken inadvertently from the proximal stomach rather than CLO, a particular problem in the presence of hiatus hernia or severe oesophagitis, a false-positive diagnosis of Barrett's oesophagus may be made in the absence of intestinal metaplasia. Increasingly the tendency now is to exclude those cases showing only fundic or cardiac type mucosa on biopsy and to classify only those with intestinal metaplasia as CLO.[14] This is partly to avoid the false-positive diagnoses, as described above, but also because it has been shown that the development of dysplasia and carcinoma is restricted to those cases with intestinal metaplasia.[12,14]

Some studies use the presence of intestinal metaplasia alone as the definition of CLO. Indeed Spechler[14] and Riddell[15] have suggested that CLO be redefined as simply intestinal metaplasia of the lower oesophagus. This has been justified in that intestinal metaplasia within either oesophageal mucosa or gastric mucosa is always pathological. However there is an inevitable problem here: if diagnostic biopsies fail to demonstrate intestinalized mucosa, that is actually present elsewhere in the CLO segment, then a diagnosis of CLO may not be made. Yet, in those cases, diagnostic biopsies have simply failed to sample the intestinalized mucosa that was actually present. Whilst this may be a problem in individual cases, it should be noted that, in our experience, all cases of traditional CLO will show intestinalized mucosa if enough biopsies are examined.[16]

There remain further difficulties in defining CLO. Endoscopic recognition of the anatomical gastro-oesophageal junction (GOJ) is not straightforward. The squamo-columnar junction (SCJ), the Z-line, usually lies within the lower oesophageal sphincter (LOS), which itself occupies the distal 3 cm of the oesophagus. Thus it is said that up to 2 cm of mucosa within the lower oesophageal sphincter may be gastric in nature. Even if one is able to accurately define the gastro-oesophageal junction, it is very difficult to accurately measure distances within the living, moving oesophagus at endoscopy.[12] The most common definition of standard CLO is the presence of at least 3 cm of CLO, with goblet cells indicative of intestinal metaplasia on biopsy (accepting that an absence of goblet cells in a biopsy from CLO may merely be a sampling error). This 3 cm definition has arisen largely because of the 2 cm anatomical variation between the true oesophago-gastric junction and the squamo-columnar junction. However this definition evidently excludes genuine short lengths of metaplastic glandular epithelium within the lower oesophagus. This is important as there is now increasing evidence that so-called short segment CLO (SSCLO) and ultrashort segment CLO (USSCLO) are probably precursor lesions in many cases of oesophageal adenocarcinoma. Indeed USSCLO has also not been tightly defined. Some regard this condition as representing small non-circumferential tongues of metaplastic mucosa in the lower oesophagus whilst others have used the term to describe intestinal metaplasia within cardiac mucosa at the squamo-columnar junction (known usually as IM of the cardia).

In 1970 an animal model of Barrett's oesophagus demonstrated oesophageal mucosal regeneration with glandular rather than squamous mucosa in the presence of chronic gastro-oesophageal reflux.[17] For many years it has been considered that the epithelial damage in the oesophagus and the glandular metaplasia are related almost exclusively to acid reflux into the oesophagus. It is recognized that CLO patients have decreased LOS pressures, increased frequency and duration of oesophageal acid exposure and delayed oesophageal acid clearance.[18] However, there is now increased interest in gastroduodenal reflux into the oesophagus and the role of bile in glandular metaplasia and neoplastic transformation. The role of the reflux of duodenal contents in the causation of oesophageal mucosal injury has been difficult to assess largely due to the lack of accurate methods to measure this. Latterly a fibre-optic system (Bilitec), using spectrophotometric measurements at a wavelength specific to bilirubin, has allowed 24-hour ambulatory monitoring of bile reflux. Using this technique clinical studies have demonstrated a graded increase in both acid and duodenogastro-oesophageal reflux from controls to patients with oesophagitis, with Barrett's patients having the highest values.[18]

Conjugated bile acids have been implicated as the component of duodenal fluid that causes mucosal injury and it is therefore of interest that the high pH environment created by proton pump inhibitors inactivates these bile acids. In keeping with this, bile reflux in non-acidic circumstances, for example in partial gastrectomy patients, does not cause mucosal injury. In the animal model of Barrett's oesophagus used by Gillen and colleagues,[19] repair of mucosal defects was by columnar epithelium in the presence of mixed acid and bile reflux mimicking Barrett's metaplasia but healing by regeneration of squamous epithelium only occurred in the presence of bile reflux alone.

Initially it was suggested that this repair of damaged oesophageal mucosa by glandular Barrett's epithelium represented ingrowth of cardiac glandular epithelium in continuity with the injured oesophageal mucosa. However the elegant animal experiments of Hennessy's group,[19,20] in which a barrier of normal squamous mucosa was left between the gastric cardia and the area of oesophageal mucosal damage, have demonstrated re-epithelialization of these defects by columnar epithelium. In the canine model,[19] oesophageal gland ducts were seen in continuity with the surface columnar epithelium, suggesting that these were the cells of origin of Barrett's mucosa. Evidence from animal models and in human CLO patients[21,22] support this concept of a multi-potential stem cell in the native glandular structures of the oesophagus. In these studies defects were produced within the segment of Barrett's mucosa and allowed to heal in the presence of acid suppression. Repair by squamous epithelium was seen despite there being no continuity with adjacent native oesophageal squamous epithelium. Wright[23] has suggested that CLO is a form of ductal migration, similar to gastric metaplasia of the duodenum and the so-called 'ulcer-associated cell lineage', arising from the oesophageal gland ducts. He proposes that there is evidence for CLO being such a glandular epithelial repair mechanism in that it actively secretes peptides that promote epithelial repair.[23] Against this is the evidence, promoted by some, that metaplasia occurs from pluripotent stem cells within the squamous mucosa of the oesophagus.[24]

There is much interest in the role of *Helicobacter pylori* (HP) in the pathogenesis of CLO and its progression to adenocarcinoma. There is an increasing body of evidence linking USSCLO (or at least that type also known as IM of the cardia) with HP infection and intestinal metaplasia elsewhere in the stomach.[25–27] Conversely, there is increasing evidence of a reciprocal relationship between HP and traditional/classical CLO and SSCLO.[28,29] It has been suggested that gastric infection, especially pangastric, with cag-A-positive strains of HP may be protective against CLO.[28] It may be therefore that the dramatic changes in the prevalence of CLO and oesophago-cardiac adenocarcinoma are related to alterations in the prevalence of gastric HP infection.[28]

It has been proposed that a crucial determinant of the predominant pathology of the upper gastro-intestinal tract, in evolutionary and epidemiological terms, is the time of acquisition of HP infection.[28] Thus, ameliorating socio-economic circumstances and the widespread use of antibiotics may account for a dramatic reduction in HP gastritis in childhood and early adulthood in Western communities over the past few decades. This, in turn, explains the proximal movement in the prevalence of gastric cancer and the increase in gastro-oesophageal reflux disease (GORD), CLO and oesophageal adenocarcinoma. Indiscriminate eradication of HP may not be a sensible strategy (at least for oesophageal disease) and there must be careful consideration of potential risks as well as benefits of HP eradication policies.[28]

HISTOPATHOLOGY

Biopsies taken from endoscopically identified CLO show a range of histological appearances, characteristically described as a patchwork of the different glandular phenotypes.[30] As described previously, some authors consider the presence of intestinal metaplasia, as represented by goblet cells, to be the defining feature of CLO. Complete intestinal metaplasia, consisting of columnar epithelium with all the features of small intestinal mucosa including goblet cells, absorptive cells, Paneth cells and endocrine cells, is relatively uncommon. Incomplete intestinal metaplasia is more common: it consists of intestinal-type goblet cells lying amongst gastric-type mucin-secreting cells. These mucin-secreting cells have been termed intermediate cells, since ultrastructurally they have features of both gastric mucous cells (apical glycoprotein granules) and intestinal absorptive cells (partially developed brush border). Detection of intestinal metaplasia can be improved by the use of alcian blue (AB) staining in addition to haematoxylin & eosin (H&E).[31] Intestinal metaplasia is not always present in biopsies from CLO and the mucosa has the features of cardiac or fundic-type gastric mucosa. Indeed it has been recently intimated that cardiac mucosa, in the upper stomach, is itself metaplastic and represents an abnormal finding associated with gastro-oesophageal reflux.[32] However it must be emphasized that this is certainly not proven and is not widely accepted at this time.

Whilst both the junctional and fundic types of mucosa may represent a biopsy taken from a hiatus hernia, certain clues may allow a probable or even definite diagnosis of glandular metaplasia in the absence of goblet cells. It is obviously important to know the site from which the biopsy has been taken. The glandular mucosa in CLO is atrophic, disorganized with a non-organoid arrangement of

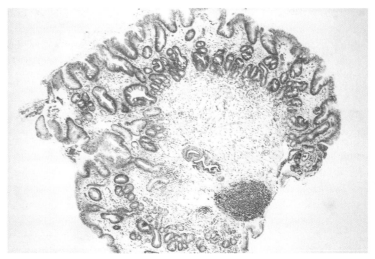

Fig. 5.3 Typical intestinalized Barrett's mucosa is present on the surface. Centrally, adjacent to a small lymphoid follicle is an oesophageal gland duct. This serves to confirm unequivocally the diagnosis of CLO.

glands when compared with true cardiac (assuming this mucosa to be physiological and not metaplastic) or fundic gastric mucosa. It characteristically shows a patchwork of the different epithelial types. The presence of native oesophageal structures, oesophageal gland ducts most commonly or alternatively submucosal glands, allow histological confirmation of the oesophageal origin of the biopsy and thus CLO (Fig. 5.3). However, our own study has shown that these structures are only present in about 15% of biopsies taken to confirm the diagnosis of CLO.[16]

MUCIN HISTOCHEMISTRY

The intermediate columnar cells of CLO may produce neutral mucin resembling normal gastric surface foveolar epithelium or acidic mucin staining positively with AB at pH 2.5. The acidic mucin is either sialomucin or sulphated mucin, which can be distinguished by high iron diamine which stains sulphomucins brown in colour. This variation in acid mucin production has been used to subdivide intestinal metaplasia (IM) into the Type II incomplete IM, in which the intermediate cells produce either neutral mucins or sialomucins, and Type III incomplete IM in which these cells also produce sulphated acidic mucins as well as the neutral and sialomucins. The presence of AB-positive intermediate cells, cells without the barrel-shaped morphology of true goblet cells, are not diagnostic of Barrett's specialized mucosa. They are also found in the mucous neck region of gastric glands and in reactive gastric epithelium.[33] Goblet cells in intestinal metaplasia produce acidic mucins that again can be either sulphated or non-sulphated.

Whilst much has been written about these characteristic mucin changes of CLO, it has to be emphasized that there is no phenotype, be it mucin biochemical or any other, that is absolutely specific to CLO. The mucin histochemistry is certainly highly distinctive for CLO but the same phenotype can be seen, admittedly less commonly, in the stomach, for instance. Thus the mucin phenotype can only be described as highly characteristic rather than pathogno-monic of CLO. It has been suggested that the presence of sulphomucins is asso-ciated with the development of dysplasia and subsequent carcinoma.[34] However the presence of these mucins is so common (57.9% of BO in one study) that they are not useful for identifying a high–risk group for screening.

SHORT SEGMENT AND ULTRA-SHORT SEGMENT CLO

An inevitable consequence of the rigid definition of CLO as greater than 3 cm of circumferential metaplastic epithelium is the exclusion of shorter lengths of CLO. However intestinal metaplasia anywhere in the oesophagus or gastric cardia is clearly pathological and there is evidence that these shorter lengths of CLO are associated with dysplasia and may progress to carcinoma.[35] SSCLO is best defined as less than 3 cm of CLO with intestinal metaplasia on biopsy whereas intestinal metaplasia in biopsies from an endoscopically normal GOJ has been referred to as USSCLO. Both of these diseases show a much higher prevalence than traditional CLO (Table 5.1).[31,36,37] Whilst patients with SSCLO report reflux symptoms more frequently than traditional CLO patients, they have less severe measurable disturbances in oesophageal motility and reflux.[36] The limited studies available suggest that dysplasia is less common in SSCLO than traditional CLO although there is evidence that SSCLO is associated with adenocarcinoma although the magnitude of risk is not known.[36,37] This is largely because the great majority of adenocarcinomas of the oesophagus are detected in patients in whom a previous diagnosis of CLO had not been made: the difficulties are compounded by the fact that advanced oesophageal carcinoma often destroys the small foci of CLO (Fig. 5.4), rendering it impossible to confirm the pre-existence of short segment disease.

There are a few studies in which the prevalence and associations of intestinal metaplasia at the endoscopically normal SCJ have been studied. It has been sug-gested that this endoscopically unsuspected IM in cardiac mucosa is a different lesion epidemiologically and pathogenetically to other forms of CLO.[25,27] Table 1 demonstrates how common this lesion is in endoscopic populations. This patient group may show a female preponderance in contrast to the male predominance seen in SSCLO and classic CLO.[26] It is associated with intestinal metaplasia and atrophy elsewhere in the stomach and with HP infection and not with gastro-oesophageal reflux disease.[26,27] This is in contrast with SSCLO, which shows the same association with gastro-oesophageal reflux as traditional CLO.

This area of oesophago-gastric pathology remains confusing most notably because of the lack of uniformity in the definitions of SSCLO and USSCLO.

Table 5.1 A comparison of the prevalence, associations and neoplastic potential of traditional CLO, short segment CLO (SSCLO) and ultra-short segment CLO (USSCLO)

	Traditional CLO	SSCLO	USSCLO
Prevalence*	1–3%	8–17%	18–36%
Association with GORD	Certain	Certain	Unlikely
Association with HP	Reciprocal	Probably reciprocal	Positive
Malignant potential	+++	++	? +

*Prevalence in endoscopic populations.

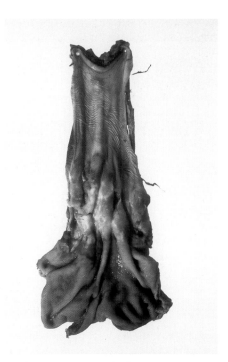

Fig. 5.4 A typical stricturing lower oesophageal adenocarcinoma. The tumour has destroyed all mucosa at the lower aspect of the oesophagus, rendering it impossible to demonstrate any pre-existing CLO. An unusual feature is the presence of a submucosal tumour nodule 10 cm proximal to the main tumour.

Clearly it is necessary for some consensus to be reached in defining these entities if useful epidemiological, pathogenetic and prognostic information is to be produced. Spechler[14] has proposed an alternative classification that does not depend upon arbitrary and imprecise endoscopic measurements. He suggests that whenever columnar epithelium is seen in the oesophagus, regardless of extent, it should be termed columnar-lined oesophagus, biopsied and then classified as demonstrated in Table 5.2.

Table 5.2 A model of CLO and cardia IM classification

	Association with GORD	*Association with adenocarcinoma*	*Endoscopic surveillance recommended*
CLO with intestinal metaplasia	Variable	Yes	Yes
CLO without intestinal metaplasia	Variable	Unlikely	Probably not
Intestinal metaplasia at GOJ	Unclear, probably not	Probable	Unclear, probably not

GORD, gastro-oesophageal reflux disease; CLO, columnar lined oesophagus; GOJ, gastro-oesophageal junction.
Source: Spechler.[14]

DYSPLASIA IN CLO

It is well recognized that there is a progression from metaplasia through dysplasia to adenocarcinoma in CLO and it is now generally accepted that the classification of neoplastic change in CLO should conform to that given in Table 5.3. The restriction of dysplasia to two grades, low (LGD) and high (HGD), is more helpful for individual patient management. The detection of pre-malignant change, dysplasia, in CLO is profoundly reliant on accurate pathology but there remain great problems with the identification of dysplasia in CLO and therefore of patients at high risk of carcinoma. First it is usually not possible to distinguish dysplasia from non-dysplastic glandular mucosa using routine endoscopic techniques.[38] HGD and adenocarcinoma can be detected in biopsies from macroscopically unremarkable Barrett's mucosa or can be associated with minimal visual abnormalities such as small erosions, plaques or polyps (Fig. 5.5).[39] There is also a sampling problem with areas of dysplasia being missed if insufficient biopsies are taken. Recommended biopsy protocols for patients being surveyed for dysplasia suggest four quadrant biopsies at 2 cm levels within the Barrett's segment as well as multiple biopsies of any macroscopic abnormality such as nodules, erosions or plaques.[15,39]

As well as the problems of the endoscopic recognition of dysplasia, there is also considerable inter-observer variation in the histological diagnosis of dysplasia, particularly for LGD.[40] As in other sites in the GI tract, dysplasia is characterized by architectural and cytological abnormalities. In LGD there is minimal architectural disturbance, nuclei are confined to the lower half of the cells and mucin production is often maintained. In HGD there is more marked architectural abnormality including villous change and cribriform glands (Fig. 5.6). Nuclear stratification is usually present throughout the whole height of the columnar cells and loss of mucin is seen. Intramucosal carcinoma is recognized by the presence of irregular groups of cells or single cells within the stroma eliciting a desmoplastic response. Whilst reasonable agreement can be achieved for the diagnosis of HGD, the main difficulty is in distinguishing LGD from reactive changes.[40] Indeed the intestinal-type glands often show marked nuclear 'activity' in contrast to the gastric-type mucosa and this has considerable propensity for the overdiagnosis of dysplasia. In particular, given the patchwork nature of CLO, the juxtaposition of 'normal' gastric-type mucosa with hyperplastic intestinal-type mucosa can trap the unwary into an overdiagnosis of dysplasia.[16] However, these hyperplastic changes are restricted to the deeper part of the gland, the proliferative zone, and normal maturation of the surface epithelial cells is seen. This is in contrast to LGD where the cytological abnormalities extend to involve the surface epithelium.

Table 5.3. The classification of neoplastic change in CLO

Negative for dysplasia
Indefinite for dysplasia
Low grade dysplasia
High grade dysplasia
Intramucosal carcinoma
Invasive adenocarcinoma

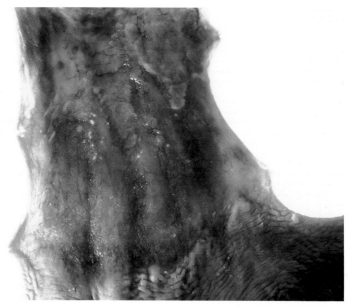

Fig. 5.5 A resection specimen demonstrating a CLO segment between the Z-line of the oesophago-gastric junction and the oesophageal squamous mucosa (above). A small nodule is just visible (at left) which showed invasive adenocarcinoma. However there was widespread 'field change' of HGD in the CLO segment and this is entirely invisible to the naked eye.

The use of an 'indefinite for dysplasia' category analogous to that used in the grading of dysplasia in inflammatory bowel disease is appropriate in those difficult borderline cases, often in the presence of active inflammation. Early re-endoscopy and multiple biopsies following treatment of the inflammation often resolve the issue. LGD is an indication for close endoscopic surveillance with multiple segmental and quadrantic biopsies.

The diagnosis of HGD in CLO is one of considerable import. Correlation of the biopsy diagnosis of HGD with the findings in subsequent oesophagectomy specimens has shown that HGD coexists with invasive adenocarcinoma in 38–64% of cases.[1,16] Thus many regard HGD as an indication for oesophagectomy and would advise that the pathological diagnosis of HGD is either corroborated by further biopsies or is confirmed by a second, preferably expert, pathologist.

ANCILLARY HISTOLOGICAL TECHNIQUES

In view of the difficulties in the diagnosis of dysplasia, many workers have sought alternative markers of high risk of progression to carcinoma, aside from morphological assessment for dysplasia. In more recent years the emphasis has been on molecular markers (*vide infra*). In this section some selected non-molecular markers will be considered. Some have postulated an increased risk of carcinoma in patients with sulphomucin expression in the intermediate cells of Barrett's mucosa but others have found no predictive value of sulphomucins for either dysplasia or malignancy.[33] Sulphated mucins within goblet cells are so

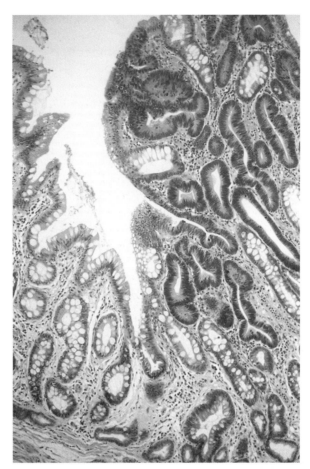

Fig. 5.6 High grade dysplasia in CLO. There is marked architectural abnormality with polypoid change, contrasting with the adjacent non-neoplastic intestinalized CLO mucosa. Elsewhere there was invasive adenocarcinoma.

common (indeed in our studies and others of traditional CLO effectively universal)[39,41,42] as to be entirely unhelpful as a marker of increased cancer risk.

One study has shown that patients with CLO and cancer were more often Lewis[a+ b-] non-secretors and blood group A than Barrett's patients without cancer and the normal population.[34] These workers also identified a subtype of intestinal metaplasia in CLO expressing sulphomucins and aberrant Le[a] antigen in goblet and columnar cells associated with a high risk of malignancy. However, this was a cross-sectional study and prospective studies are needed to further evaluate these findings. Expression of Glut1, the human erythrocyte transporter, has been suggested to demonstrate absolute specificity for adenocarcinoma in CLO but it has a relatively low sensitivity.[43]

MOLECULAR PATHOLOGY

The molecular biology of the progression of CLO through the metaplasia–dysplasia–carcinoma sequence has not been studied to the same extent as the analogous colorectal adenoma–carcinoma sequence. Nevertheless progress has been made and we are starting to be able to produce a reasonable model of the molecular events that underpin the progression of this neoplastic sequence of CLO (Fig. 5.7).[24,44] Elucidation of events at the molecular level will aid the clinical management of CLO, for example by identifying markers of high risk of progression to carcinoma and of prognosis in patients who have already developed adenocarcinoma. Research into the molecular biology of the CLO neoplastic sequence has concentrated on five main areas: cell cycle abnormalities and apoptosis, oncogenic mutations and over-expressions, cell adhesion, DNA instability and the role of proteolytic enzymes and angiogenesis in invasion.[24]

The growth rate of a tissue is determined by the balance between proliferation and apoptosis.[45] Cells with DNA damage that cannot be repaired are usually eliminated by apoptosis. Those that survive continue to proliferate, allowing propagation of genetic defects.[46] Changes are seen in the distribution of the proliferative zone of the crypt during the metaplasia–dysplasia–carcinoma sequence of CLO.[47] In dysplasia the proliferative zone expands from the glandular zone to the luminal surface indicating disruption in the control of proliferation.[48,49] Conversely apoptosis is reduced in dysplasia and carcinoma, perhaps because of over-expression of bcl-2, resulting in a cell survival advantage in dysplasia and carcinoma.[49,50] Our studies have demonstrated the utility of the assessment of both proliferative activity and apoptosis in the differentiation of non-neoplastic mucosa and dysplasia, especially when analysing the surface mucosa.[49] Perhaps semi-automation of such techniques offers some hope for the non-subjective demonstration of dysplasia in CLO.[49,51]

Expression of p53, the protein of the tumour suppressor gene found on chromosome 17p, which is of critical importance in the promotion of apoptosis in cells with mutant DNA, is thought to be disrupted early in the metaplasia–dysplasia–carcinoma sequence through gene loss, mutation or over-expression.[44]

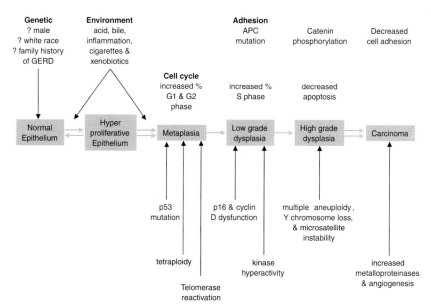

Fig. 5.7 A 'Vogelsteinogram' of the molecular and pathogenetic factors in the progression of the neoplastic sequence of CLO.

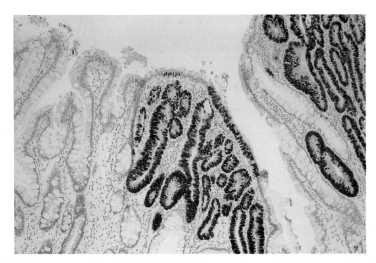

Fig. 5.8 p53 over-expression in HGD of CLO in the same focus of HGD demonstrated in Fig. 5.6. The dramatic nuclear positivity is only seen in dysplastic mucosa and not in the adjacent intestinalized but non-neoplastic CLO mucosa.

Studies of the expression of p53 in CLO and associated adenocarcinoma using immunocytochemistry have shown that p53 over-expression is relatively specific for HGD (Fig. 5.8) and adenocarcinoma but is of low sensitivity (around 50–60%).[52,53] Others have suggested that p53 protein accumulation, as detected by immunohistochemistry, has a higher predictive value for malignant progression than the presence of LGD and/or mucosa indefinite for dysplasia, demonstrated morphologically.[54] We would maintain that, of all markers currently available to the routine laboratory, p53 is probably the most useful in terms of substantiating a diagnosis of HGD and/or adenocarcinoma although low sensitivity remains a problem.

Controversies surround the importance, in CLO neoplasia, of the oncogene c-erbB2, which produces a 185 kDa Type 1 growth factor receptor with similarities to Epithelial Growth Factor Receptor (EGFR) and with tyrosine kinase activity. Over-expression of c-erbB2 appears to be a late event in the development of some adenocarcinomas arising from CLO,[55] and has been correlated with poor survival,[45] whilst in another study over-expression predicted a favourable response to chemotherapy.[56] The APC gene, which maps to chromosome 5q21, is a tumour suppressor gene involved in the control of growth and proliferation of epithelial cells, whose malfunction is central to the adenoma–carcinoma sequence of colorectal cancer. Studies have demonstrated loss of heterozygosity (LOH) for APC occurring in adenocarcinoma arising in CLO, in adjacent dysplastic columnar epithelium and also in adjacent non-dysplastic metaplastic epithelium.[57,58] However APC appears to have a more limited role in oesophageal adenocarcinoma development than in colorectal carcinogenesis. Other tumour suppressor gene loci have also been demonstrated to show LOH in Barrett's cancers, the highest rates (all above 50%) being for VHL (chromosome 3p), CDKN2 (chromosome 9p), Rb (chromosome 13q) and DCC (chromosome 18q).[24,59]

Cell adhesion abnormalities appear to be pivotal to the neoplastic progression of CLO (Fig. 5.7). Loss of membranous E-cadherin expression occurs in metaplasia: in intestinal type Barrett's mucosa, 25% of cases show a reduction in immunoreactivity,[60] and in dysplasia staining becomes further reduced and disorganized.[61,62] Catenin expression shows similar alterations in the progression of CLO through dysplasia to carcinoma.[62] Nuclear translocation of β-catenin and γ-catenin, in dysplasia and early carcinoma, may well be a critical step in neoplastic progression, the nuclear localization of these proteins having direct effects on transcription (Fig. 5.9).[62] Reduced E-cadherin expression in CLO tumours has been shown to correlate with shorter survival and expression of catenins may offer similar prognostic information.[63] CD44 is also involved in cell–cell adhesion in addition to other functions such as lymphocyte homing.[64] Different splice variants have been identified in tumourigenesis, and these may provide diagnostic and prognostic information in certain cancers.[65] Two isoforms, CD44H and CD44v3, have been studied in CLO and associated adenocarcinomas: CD44H is expressed in proliferating areas of normal squamous epithelium and CLO, increasing in dysplasia and adenocarcinoma.[66] CD44v3, expressed in squamous epithelium but not CLO or dysplasia, is also expressed in adenocarcinoma and may play a role in tumourigenesis.[66]

There appears to be relatively good correlation between high grade dysplasia, as diagnosed by routine pathology, and aneuploidy, usually determined by flow

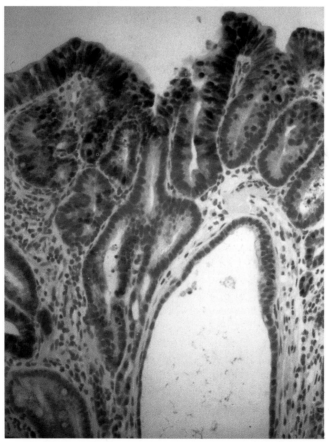

Fig. 5.9 Immunohistochemistry demonstrating nuclear translocation of ß-catenin in high grade dysplasia in CLO (well seen in the dysplastic surface mucosa). The protein translocation has direct effects on transcription and is probably a critical step in the neoplastic progression.

cytometry.[24] Nevertheless, as with all other 'markers of neoplastic change', the role of flow cytometry in the diagnosis of neoplasia in CLO remains unproven. Whilst we continue to understand more of the molecular events that lead to malignancy in the oesophagus, none of these 'markers' have progressed enough to allow their confident usage in the routine management of CLO patients: all should be currently considered experimental only.[7]

CYTOLOGY

Given the problems with the histological diagnosis of CLO, and of dysplasia in particular, can cytology provide any diagnostic aid? Brush cytology of the oesophagus at endoscopy can confirm the presence of glandular epithelium and goblet cells, and thus of CLO, but it is neither as sensitive nor as specific as histology.[67] Balloon cytology has been evaluated as a non-endoscopic screening technique for CLO. However one study has shown that, of 10 patients with known CLO, none showed goblet cells on cytology.[68] Thus we cannot recommend cytology for the identification of CLO.

The use of cytology for the assessment of dysplasia in patients known to have CLO has been addressed by several studies. As the differentiation between HGD and invasive carcinoma is essentially an architectural one, one would not expect to be able to distinguish these using cytology alone and this is borne out in practice.[69] Nevertheless, in theory, it is possible to sample a larger area using brush cytology, compared with biopsy, and it has been intimated that it might be useful in identifying macroscopically inconspicuous areas of dysplasia.[70] Cost is an important consideration in surveillance programmes and a sixfold reduction in cost has been demonstrated when using non-endoscopic balloon cytology instead of endoscopic techniques to diagnose dysplasia in CLO.[71] In that study, balloon cytology detected 80% of patients with HGD/carcinoma when sufficient material was obtained (83% of patients) although sensitivity for LGD was much lower (25%).[71] Cytology may well have a role in the surveillance of CLO patients, especially if the non-endoscopic balloon methods can be combined with sensitive molecular analyses for demonstrating early neoplastic change.

NATURAL HISTORY OF DYSPLASIA AND THE MANAGEMENT CONTROVERSY

The progression of LGD through HGD to invasive adenocarcinoma is now well recognized but the time scale of this sequence shows marked patient-to-patient variation. In one prospective study, five out of 50 CLO patients developing adenocarcinoma showed dysplasia on biopsy prior to identification of invasive carcinoma but the time interval between the demonstration of LGD and carcinoma varied from 1.5 to 4 years.[72] In another study, the mean time for progression of indefinite/LGD to HGD was 29 months in seven patients.[33] However, there is also some evidence to suggest that low grade/indefinite dysplasia can regress with follow-up biopsies being negative for dysplasia.[73] In a 'screened' population of CLO patients with LGD, only 13% progressed to HGD or adenocarcinoma.[74] However, this may simply reflect sampling error or, in some cases, reflect the fact that some cases merely represent florid reactive or inflammatory change rather than a true neoplastic process. The consensus with regard to the management of LGD (and of mucosa indefinite for dysplasia) reflects this problem and recommends early and regular follow-up endoscopy and repeat biopsy following anti-reflux and antacid therapy.

HGD is much more strongly associated with carcinoma. In one study progression from HGD to cancer in five patients required, on average, 14 months or, expressed another way, about 50% of patients with HGD will develop adenocarcinoma during a 5 year follow-up period.[33,75] Against this, however, are described cases in which HGD has been present for considerable periods of time without progression to cancer, in some cases at least 4 years.[72] Sampling error remains a problem in the diagnosis of HGD and invasive carcinoma.

A meta-analysis of published reports of surgical resection for HGD in CLO included 119 patients who underwent oesophagectomy with a pre-operative diagnosis of HGD only.[76] Pathological examination of the resection specimens showed 47% of these harboured foci of invasive carcinoma. In individual series, the coexistence of biopsy-diagnosed HGD with frank adenocarcinoma, diagnosed at the time of resection, varies from 38% to 64%.[16] This is a powerful reason why many centres now recommend surgical resection of the oesophagus when a corroborated diagnosis of HGD is made on biopsy. The accuracy of the biopsy diagnosis of HGD is critical: many would advise that the pathological diagnosis of HGD is either authenticated by further biopsies or confirmed by a second, preferably expert, pathologist.

In support of early operative intervention for HGD in CLO, carcinomas detected at the time of resection show much earlier stage (the meta-analysis showed 73% of the invasive carcinomas to be stage 1), in marked comparison to the much more advanced stage of unselected populations of Barrett's cancer patients.[76] The decision to operate depends critically on the patient's age and co-morbidity. If these are adverse, then new ablative techniques, such as laser and photodynamic therapy, are available which provide valid, non-surgical alternative treatments.

TREATMENT AND ASSOCIATED HISTOLOGICAL CHANGES

In theory eradication of the metaplastic columnar epithelium should result in the elimination of the associated increased risk of neoplasia. Thus there is increasing interest in various techniques for the treatment and ablation of Barrett's mucosa and histopathologists will be increasingly involved in the assessment of response to these treatments. These methods include medical and surgical therapies aimed at normalizing the oesophageal pH, mainly proton pump inhibitors (PPIs) and anti-reflux surgical procedures, and direct ablative techniques including laser ablation and photodynamic therapy (PDT).[77,78] Photodynamic therapy is theoretically more specific than laser therapy, particularly for dysplasia, because the sensitizer used can be selected to be specifically absorbed by epithelial cells with the resultant specific destruction of the CLO.[77] Laser therapy, on the other hand, is critically dependent upon the depth of tissue destruction: it is important for oesophageal submucosal glands and their ducts to survive to allow squamous regeneration in the presence of acid suppression (usually by PPIs).[20,78]

Squamous re-epithelialization is seen in biopsies following treatment with

PPIs alone, or in combination with anti-reflux surgery, laser ablation and PDT (Fig. 5.10).[22] Endoscopically, islands of squamous epithelium are seen within the CLO and, if biopsies are taken to avoid these macroscopic islands, microscopic foci of squamous re-epithelialization are seen. These show different histological patterns, suggesting varying underlying mechanisms. These include encroachment of squamous epithelium over glandular mucosa adjacent to the SCJ and the presence of islands of superficial squamous epithelium within the Barrett's mucosa, often in continuity with underlying oesophageal gland ducts.[22] A third interesting pattern of squamous re-epithelialization is seen most strikingly following laser therapy and PDT.[22] Squamous metaplasia may be seen within Barrett's glands giving a histological appearance akin to that seen in immature squamous metaplasia in the uterine cervix. These findings support the concept of a multi-potential stem cell within the oesophagus, in oesophageal gland ducts capable of differentiating to CLO and in CLO capable of differentiating to squamous mucosa.[22,77] The presence of these cells at least suggests that we have the ability to convert pre-neoplastic CLO glands to mature squamous mucosa, particularly in an anacid environment.

Currently, however, PPI therapy, anti-reflux surgery, laser therapy and PDT very rarely result in complete squamous re-epithelialization. Many consider partial regression to be an inadequate endpoint, when considering the efficacy of treatment in terms of prevention of neoplastic progression.[79] Furthermore surface squamous mucosa overlying glandular mucosa of CLO-type is now a well recognized phenomenon (Fig. 5.10).[15,21,22,80] One may speculate that the buried Barrett's epithelium may be protected from the toxic stimuli within the oesophageal lumen with resulting reduction in cell proliferation leading to a reduced neoplastic risk.[22] However such buried glandular mucosa has also been seen following treatment of dysplastic CLO, with squamous re-epithelialization overlying dysplastic glandular mucosa.[22,77] This is of considerable concern because such treatment may result in the concealment of, ultimately, advanced malignancy: these findings emphasize the need for histological confirmation of squamous re-epithelialization with adequately deep biopsies.[22]

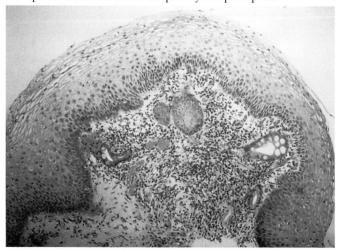

Fig. 5.10 Squamous re-epithelialization in a CLO patient treated with laser ablation. Barrett's glands survive beneath the surface squamous mucosa although the central gland has itself undergone squamous epithelialization.

The recognition of CLO, and particularly of dysplastic CLO, as a pre-malignant condition appears to provide an opportunity for identification of patients at risk of developing adenocarcinoma of the oesophagus or gastric cardia. However several points need to be considered. What is the risk of progression from CLO to adenocarcinoma? Does identification of these patients in the context of a surveillance programme, rather than as a result of symptoms, prolong survival? Is the potential surveillance test acceptable to the patient and is an effective treatment available if dysplasia or malignancy is detected? Is surveillance cost-effective on a population basis?

Various studies quote the incidence of adenocarcinoma arising in CLO as between 1:100 and 1:200 patient years with dysplasia as a marker of increased risk.[5,6,74] In a cohort of 166 patients in whom the diagnosis of CLO had been established with a total follow-up of 1440 patient years and mean follow-up of 9.3 years, eight patients developed oesophageal adenocarcinoma, seven of whom were symptomatic whilst one carcinoma was detected at endoscopic follow-up for reflux treatment.[6] The study demonstrated length of CLO and peptic ulceration to be increased risk factors for carcinoma.[6] In a UK study of a 10 year surveillance programme, only one case of adenocarcinoma was detected solely as the result of the programme (379 endoscopies) with another two patients being identified due to increasing dysphagia requiring additional endoscopies.[81] All three of these patients had long segment CLO or a stricture at the initial endoscopy. The authors comment that 'our screening programme resulted in the identification of only one patient with asymptomatic carcinoma but resulted in an additional workload equivalent to one month's work by our entire endoscopy unit. This leads us to question the value of continuing this programme'.[81] Wright et al[82] reported a more favourable experience with the detection of six carcinomas in a group of 166 patients undergoing annual surveillance. They also reported a less advanced stage of disease in the surveyed population compared with carcinomas developing in an unsurveyed control group,[82] a finding confirmed by others.[83]

There is some evidence that surveillance-detected oesophageal adenocarcinomas have a lower pathological stage and a better clinical outcome than tumours presenting symptomatically. However, the fact that the incidence of adenocarcinoma in Barrett's patients is relatively low and that adenocarcinoma is an uncommon cause of death in these patients raises the question of whether surveillance of all CLO patients is cost-effective. Only those individuals fit enough to undergo oesophagectomy, or perhaps other ablative-type therapies, should be surveyed. Reduction in cost may be achieved by targeting surveillance at higher risk groups, for example those with long segments of CLO, strictures or ulcers within the CLO or dysplasia on initial biopsy. Annual endoscopies may not be required and a prospective study has found that no patient with non-dysplastic CLO developed HGD or carcinoma in less than 2 years from initial diagnosis, suggesting that 2 yearly surveillance should be sufficient.[74] Cheaper surveillance tests, such as non-endoscopic balloon cytology rather than endoscopy with biopsy, are also being assessed[71] but the sensitivity and specificity of these tests is still being evaluated.

All these strategies require the identification of patients with CLO before they can be considered for surveillance. It is of considerable concern that, in an unselected patient population, only about 5% of lower oesophageal adenocarcinomas occur in patients already known to have CLO.[1,85] In the population there remains a huge reservoir of patients, who, because they have developed CLO in response to their acid reflux and are thus largely asymptomatic, do not come to the attention of the medical fraternity until they develop dysphagia, that harbinger symptom of established, and often late stage, adenocarcinoma. This suggests that CLO surveillance can only ever hope to achieve a reduction in mortality from oesophageal adenocarcinoma of about 5%. Nevertheless there remains a large patient group with confirmed CLO who demand a consensus management strategy. The surveillance debate will continue but histopathologists will inevitably be expected to examine greater numbers of quadrantic and segmental biopsies taken from Barrett's segments as part of surveillance programmes.

KEY POINTS

1. Barrett's oesophagus has been recognized in recent years as a major risk factor for the development of oesophageal adenocarcinoma.
2. Currently oesophageal carcinoma has a poor prognosis when presenting symptomatically. Hence surveillance of Barrett's oesophagus patients with the aim of early detection has been proposed.
3. Histopathology remains the key method of detection of Barrett's oesophagus and progression to adenocarcinoma.
4. However, advances in the understanding of the molecular mechanisms involved in the progression to adenocarcinoma may result in the development of markers for early stage neoplasia.
5. Cytology may have a role in the surveillance of columnar lined oesophagus (CLO) patients, but lacks the sensitivity and specificity of histological techniques for early diagnosis.
6. Novel medical therapies for the treatment of Barrett's mucosa are being investigated, as are novel techniques for the ablation of the metaplastic columnar epithelium.
7. Evidence suggests that surveillance of CLO patients can only hope to reduce mortality from oesophageal carcinoma by about 5%, and the surveillance debate continues.

REFERENCES

1. Cameron AJ. Epidemiology of columnar-lined esophagus and adenocarcinoma. Gastroenterol Clin N Am 1997; 26: 487–493
2. Prach AT, MacDonald TA, Hopwood DA, Johnston DA. Increasing incidence of Barrett's oesophagus: education, enthusiasm, or epidemiology? Lancet 1997; 350: 933 (Letter)
3. Blot W, Devesa SS, Fraumeni JF. Continuing climb in rates of esophageal adenocarcinoma: an update. JAmMedAssoc 1993; 270: 1320 (Letter)
4. Pera M, Cameron AJ, Trastek VF, Carpenter HA, Zinsmeister AR. Increasing incidence of adenocarcinoma of the esophagus and esophagogastric junction. Gastroenterology 1993; 104: 510–513
5. van der Veen AH, Dees J, Blankensteijn JD, van Blankenstein M. Adenocarcinoma in Barrett's oesophagus: an overrated risk. Gut 1989; 30: 14–18

6. van der Burgh A, Hop WCJ, van Blankenstein M. Oesophageal cancer is an uncommon cause of death in patients with Barrett's oesophagus. Gut 1996; 39: 5–8

7. Riddell RH. Early detection of neoplasia of the esophagus and gastroesophageal junction. Am J Gastroenterol 1996; 91: 853–863

8. Drewitz DJ, Sampliner RE, Garewal HS. The incidence of adenocarcinoma in Barrett's esophagus: a prospective study of 170 patients followed 4.8 years. Am J Gastroenterol 1997; 92: 212–215

9. Barrett NR. Chronic peptic ulcer of the oesophagus and 'oesophagitis'. Br J Surg 1950; 38: 175–182

10. Bosher LH, Taylor FH. Heterotopic gastric mucosa in the esophagus with ulceration and stricture formation. J Thoracic Surg 1951; 21: 1561–1578

11. Morson BC, Belcher JR. Adenocarcinoma of the esophagus and ectopic gastric mucosa. Br J Cancer 1952; 6: 127–130

12. Spechler SJ, Goyal RK. The columnar-lined esophagus, intestinal metaplasia, and Norman Barrett. Gastroenterology 1996; 110: 614–621

13. Barrett NR. The lower oesophagus lined by columnar epithelium. Surgery 1957; 41: 881–894

14. Spechler SJ. The columnar-lined esophagus. History, terminology, and clinical issues. Gastroenterol Clin N Am 1997; 26: 455–466

15. Riddell RH. The biopsy diagnosis of gastroesophageal reflux disease, 'carditis', and Barrett's esophagus, and sequelae of therapy. Am J Surg Pathol 1996; 20: S31–S50

16. Shepherd NA, Biddlestone LR. The histopathology and cytopathology of Barrett's oesophagus. In Manek S (Ed.) Continuing Professional Development Bulletin Cellular Pathology. Vol. 1. London: Rila Publications, 1999; 39–44

17. Bremner CG, Lynch VP, Ellis PH. Barrett's esophagus: congenital or acquired? An experimental study of esophageal mucosal regeneration in the dog. Surgery 1970; 68: 209–216

18. Vaezi MF, Richter JE. Bile reflux in columnar lined esophagus. Gastroenterol Clin N Am 1997; 26: 565–582

19. Gillen P, Keeling P, Byrne PJ, West AB, Hennessy TPJ. Experimental columnar metaplasia in the canine oesophagus. Br J Surg 1998; 75: 113–115

20. Li H, Walsh TN, O'Dowd G et al. Mechanisms of columnar metaplasia and squamous regeneration in experimental Barrett's esophagus. Surgery 1994; 115: 176–181

21. Berenson MM, Johnson TD, Markowitz NR, Buchi KN, Samowitz WS. Restoration of squamous mucosa after ablation of Barrett's oesophageal epithelium. Gastroenterology 1993; 104: 1686–1691

22. Biddlestone LR, Barham CP, Wilkinson SP, Barr H, Shepherd NA. The histopathology of treated Barrett's oesophagus: squamous re-epithelialisation following acid suppression, laser and photodynamic therapy. Am J Surg Pathol 1998; 22: 239–245

23. Wright NA. Migrations of the ductular elements of gut-associated glands gives clues to the histogenesis of structures associated with responses to acid hypersecretory state: the origins of 'gastric metaplasia' in the duodenum of the specialised mucosa of Barrett's esophagus and of pseudopyloric metaplasia. Yale J Biol Med 1996; 6: 147–153

24. Jankowski JA, Wright NA, Meltzer SJ et al. Molecular evolution of the metaplasia-dysplasia-adenocarcinoma sequence in the esophagus. Am J Pathol 1999; 154: 975–984

25. Morales TG, Sampliner RE, Bhattacharyya A. Intestinal metaplasia of the gastric cardia. Am J Gastroenterol 1997; 92: 414–418

26. Goldblum JR, Vicari JJ, Falk GW et al. Inflammation and intestinal metaplasia of the gastric cardia: the role of gastroesophageal reflux and *H. pylori* infection. Gastroenterology 1998; 114: 633–639

27. Hacklesberger A, Gunther T, Schultze V et al. Intestinal metaplasia at the gastro-oesophageal junction: *Helicobacter pylori* gastritis or gastro-oesophageal reflux disease? Gut 1998; 43: 17–21

28. Blaser MJ. *Helicobacter pylori* and gastric diseases. Br Med J 1998; 316: 1507–1510

29. Henihan RDJ, Stuart RC, Nolan N et al. Barrett's esophagus and the presence of *Helicobacter pylori*. Am J Gastroenterol 1998; 93: 542–546

30. Appelman HD. Barrett's oesophagus — morphologic considerations. In Zuidema G, Orringer M (Eds) Shackelford's Surgery of the Alimentary Tract, 4th edn. New York: WB Saunders 1996; 244–259

31. Nandurkar S, Talley NJ, Martin CJ, Ng THK, Adams S. Short segment Barrett's oesophagus: prevalence, diagnosis and associations. Gut 1997; 40: 710–715

32. Oberg S, Peters JH, DeMeester TR et al. Inflammation and specialised intestinal metaplasia of cardiac mucosa is a manifestation of gastroesophageal reflux disease. Ann Surg 1997; 226: 522–530

33. Haggitt RC. Barrett's esophagus, dysplasia, and adenocarcinoma. Hum Pathol 1994; 25: 982–993

34. Torrado J, Ruiz B, Garay J et al. Blood group phenotypes, sulfomucins, and *Helicobacter pylori* in Barrett's esophagus. Am J Surg Pathol 1997; 21: 1023–1029

35. Sharma P, Morales TG, Bhattacharyya A, Garewal HS, Sampliner RE. Dysplasia in short-segment Barrett's esophagus: a prospective 3-year follow-up. Am J Gastroenterol 1997; 92: 2012–2016

36. Donahue D, Navab F. Significance of short-segment Barrett's esophagus. J Clin Gastroenterol 1997; 25: 480–484

37. Weston AP, Krmpotich PT, Cherian R, Dixon A, Topalosvki M. Prospective long-term endoscopic and histological follow up of short segment Barrett's esophagus: comparison with traditional long segment Barrett's esophagus. Am J Gastroenterol 1997; 92: 407–413

38. Levine DS, Haggitt RC, Blount PL et al. An endoscopic biopsy protocol can differentiate high-grade dysplasia from early adenocarcinoma in Barrett's esophagus. Gastroenterology 1993; 105: 40–50

39. Levine DS. Management of dysplasia in the columnar-lined esophagus. Gastroenterol Clin N Am 1997; 26: 613–634

40. Reid BJ, Haggitt RC, Rubin CE et al. Observer variation in the diagnosis of dysplasia in Barrett's esophagus. Hum Pathol 1988; 19: 166–178

41. Gore S, Healey CJ, Sutton R et al. The regression of columnar lined (Barrett's) oesophagus with continuous omeprazole therapy. Aliment Pharmacol Therap 1993; 7: 623–628

42. Wilkinson SP, Biddlestone L, Gore S, Shepherd NA. Regression of columnar lined (Barrett's) oesophagus with omeprazole 40 mg daily — results of five years of continuous therapy. Aliment Pharmacol Therap 1999; 13: 1005–1209

43. Younes M, Lechago LV, Somoano JR et al. Wide expression of the human erythrocyte glucose transporter Glut1 in human cancers. Cancer Res 1996; 56: 1164–1167

44. Reid B, Barrett M, Galipeau P et al. Barrett's esophagus: ordering the events that lead to cancer. Eur J Cancer Prev 1996; 5: 57–65

45. Jankowski J, Dover R. Cell proliferation, differentiation and cell death in epithelial cells of the oesophagus; a critical review of biological markers and their applications to research and diagnosis. Gullet 1993; 3: 1–15

46. Bellamy C, Malcomson R., Harrison D, Wyllie A. Cell death in health and disease: the biology and regulation of apoptosis. Sem Cancer Biol 1995; 6: 3–16

47. Gillen P, McDermott M, Grehan D, Hourihane DO'B, Hennessy TPJ. Proliferating cell nuclear antigen in the assessment of Barrett's mucosa. Br J Surg 1994; 81: 1766–1768

48. Hong MK, Laskin WB, Herman BE et al. Expansion of the Ki-67 proliferative compartment correlates with degree of dysplasia in Barrett's esophagus. Cancer 1995; 75: 423–429

49. Whittles CE, Biddlestone LR, Burton A et al. Apoptotic and proliferative activity in the neoplastic progression of Barrett's oesophagus: a comparative study. J Pathol 1999; 187: 535–540

50. Katada N, Hinder R, Smyrk T et al. Apoptosis is inhibited early in the dysplasia-carcinoma sequence of Barrett esophagus. Arch Surg 1997; 132: 728–733

51. Polkowski W, Baak J, van Lanschot J et al. Clinical decision making in Barrett's oesophagus can be supported by computerized immunoquantitation and morphometry of features associated with proliferation and differentiation. J Pathol 1998; 184: 161–168

52. Flejou JF, Potet F, Muzeau F et al. Overexpression of p53 protein in Barrett's syndrome with malignant transformation. J Clin Pathol 1993; 46: 330–333

53. Hardwick RH, Shepherd NA, Moorghen M, Newcombe PV, Alderson D. Adenocarcinoma arising in Barrett's oesophagus: evidence for the participation of p53 dysfunction in the dysplasia/carcinoma sequence. Gut 1994; 35: 764–768

54. Younes M, Ertan A, Lechago LV et al. p53 protein accumulation is a specific marker of malignant potential in Barrett's metaplasia. Dig Dis Sci 1997; 42: 697–680

55. Hardwick RH, Shepherd NA, Moorghen M, Newcomb PV, Alderson D. c-erbB-2 overexpression in the dysplasia/carcinoma sequence of Barrett's oesophagus. J Clin Pathol 1995; 48: 129–132

56. Duhaylongsod FG, Gottfried MR, Ingehart JD, Vaughn AL, Wolfe WG. The significance of c-erb B-2 and p53 immunoreactivity in patients with adenocarcinoma of the esophagus. Ann Surg 1995; 221: 677–684

57. Boynton RF, Blount PL, Yin J et al. Loss of heterozygosity involving the APC and MCC genetic loci occurs in the majority of human esophageal cancers. Proc Natl Acad Sci USA 1992; 89: 3385–3387

58. Zhuang Z, Vortmeyer AO, Mark EJ et al. Barrett's esophagus: metaplastic cells with loss of heterozygosity at the APC gene locus are precursors to invasive adenocarcinoma. Cancer Res 1996; 56: 1961–1964

59. Dolan K, Garde J, Gosney J et al. Allelotype analysis of oesophageal adenocarcinoma: loss of heterozygosity occurs at multiple sites. Br J Cancer 1998; 78: 950–957

60. Jankowski JA, Newham PM, Kandemir O et al. Differential expression of E-cadherin in normal, metaplastic and dysplastic oesophageal mucosa: a putative biomarker. Int J Oncol 1994; 4: 441–448

61. Bongiorno PF, Al-Kasspooles M, Lee SW et al. E-cadherin expression in primary and metastatic thoracic neoplasms and in Barrett's oesophagus. Br J Cancer 1995; 71: 166–172

62. Bailey T, Biddlestone L, Shepherd N et al. Altered cadherin and catenin complexes in the Barrett's esophagus–dysplasia–adenocarcinoma sequence: correlation with disease progression and dedifferentiation. Am J Pathol 1998; 52: 135–144

63. Krishnadath KK, Tilanus HW, van Blankenstein M et al. Reduced expression of the cadherin-catenin complex in oesophageal adenocarcinoma correlates with poor prognosis. J Pathol 1997; 182: 331–338

64. Shimiziu Y, van Seventer G, Siraganian R, Wahl L, Shaw S. Dual role of the CD44 molecule in T-cell adhesion and activation. J Immunol 1989; 143: 2457–2463

65. Matsumura Y, Tarin D. Significance of CD44 gene products for cancer diagnosis and disease evaluation. Lancet 1992; 340: 1053–1058

66. Castella E, Ariza A, Fernandez-Vasalo A, Roca X, Ojanguren I. Expression of CD44H and CD44v3 in normal esophagus, Barrett mucosa and esophageal carcinoma. J Clin Pathol 1996; 49: 489–492

67. Wang HH, Sovie S, Zeroogian JM et al. Value of cytology in detecting intestinal metaplasia and associated dysplasia at the gastroesophageal junction. Hum Pathol 1997; 28: 465–471

68. Fennerty MB, DiTomasso J, Morales TG et al. Screening for Barrett's oesophagus by balloon cytology. Am J Gastroenterol 1995; 90: 1230–1232

69. Alexander JA, Jones SM, Smith CJ et al. Usefulness of cytopathology and histology in the evaluation of Barrett's esophagus in a community hospital. Gastrointest Endoscopy 1997; 46: 318–320

70. Antonioli DA, Wang HH. Morphology of Barrett's esophagus and Barrett's-associated dysplasia and adenocarcinoma. Gastroenterol Clin N Am 1997; 26: 495–506

71. Falk GW, Chittajallu R, Goldblum JR et al. Surveillance of patients with Barrett's esophagus for dysplasia and cancer with balloon cytology. Gastroenterology 1997; 112: 1787–1797

72. Hameeteman W, Tytgat GNJ, Houthoff HJ, van den Tweel JG. Barrett's esophagus: development of dysplasia and adenocarcinoma. Gastroenterology 1989; 96: 1249–1256

73. Hamilton SR, Smith RRL. The relationship between columnar epithelial dysplasia and invasive adenocarcinoma arising in Barrett's oesophagus. Am J Clin Pathol 1987; 87: 301–312

74. Katz D, Rothstein R, Schned A et al. The development of dysplasia and adenocarcinoma during endoscopic surveillance of Barrett's esophagus. Am J Gastroenterol 1998; 93: 536–541

75. Reid BJ, Blount PL, Rubin CE et al. Predictors of progression to malignancy in Barrett's esophagus: endoscopic, histologic and flow cytometric follow-up of a cohort. Gastroenterology 1992; 102: 1212–1219

76. Ferguson MK, Naunheim KS. Resection for Barrett's mucosa with high grade dysplasia: implications for prophylactic photodynamic therapy. J Thoracic Cardiovasc Surg 1997; 114: 824–829

77. Barr H, Shepherd NA, Dix A et al. Eradication of high-grade dysplasia in columnar lined (Barrett's) oesophagus by photodynamic therapy with endogenously generated protoporphyrin IX. Lancet 1996; 348: 584–585

78. Barham CP, Jones RL, Biddlestone LR et al. Photothermal laser ablation of Barrett's oesophagus: endoscopic and histological evidence of squamous re-epithelialisation. Gut 1997; 41: 281–284

79. Sharma P, Morales TG, Bhattacharyya A, Garewal HS, Sampliner RE. Squamous islands in Barrett's esophagus: what lies underneath? Am J Gastroenterol 1998; 93: 332–335

80. Skinner DB, Walther BC, Riddell RH et al. Barrett's esophagus. Comparison of benign and malignant cases. Ann Surg 1983; 198: 554–566

81. Macdonald CE, Wicks AC, Playford RJ. Ten years experience of screening patients with Barrett's oesophagus in a university teaching hospital. Gut 1997; 41: 303–307

82. Wright TA, Gray MR, Morris AI et al. Cost effectiveness of detecting Barrett's cancer. Gut 1996; 39: 574–579

83. van Sandick JW, van Lanschot JJB, Kuiken BW et al. Impact of endoscopic biopsy surveillance of Barrett's oesophagus on pathological stage and clinical outcome in Barrett's oesophagus. Gut 1998; 43: 216–222

84. Brown CM, Jones R, Shirazi T, Codling B, Valori RM. Prior diagnosis of Barrett's oesophagus is rare in patients with oesophageal carcinoma. Gut 1996; 38 (Abstract)

6

X-ray micro-computed tomography using synchrotron radiation

Tohoru Takeda Yuji Itai

INTRODUCTION

Imaging plays an important role as a research tool in medicine and biology. In particular, conventional X-ray computed tomography (CT), which was developed by Hounsfield in 1979,[1] is an indispensable modality for diagnosing many kinds of disease in clinical practice. Currently, X-ray CT is mainly used to demonstrate morphological and vessel structures using iodine contrast agents. In addition, the recent development of helical X-ray CT has made it possible to obtain information on the three-dimensional morphological structure of various organs, vessels and bronchi. For functional imaging, the cerebral blood flow can be estimated using stable xenon inhalation.[2,3] However, the spatial resolution of clinically used CT systems has to be more than 300 μm owing to the limited X-ray dose advisable for patients.

Monochromatic X-ray CT with synchrotron radiation (SR) is being developed for the analysis of the fine structure of biological material in scientific research because it has an adequate X-ray flux and the energy spectrum can be fine-tuned for the visualization of the spatial distribution of specific elements.

In 1983, Grodzins proposed synchrotron radiation as an alternative X-ray source for CT.[4,5] Biomedical experiments have imaged the dog heart[6] and human lymph node[7] using iodine contrast material, and also the human finger bone[8] and a live rat skull.[9] Currently, it is possible to obtain very fine images of bony structures with a spatial resolution in the um range.[10-14] A highly sensitive SR X-ray CT system has been developed for revealing a map of low and intermediate Z-elements for neurological diagnosis[15-17] and high Z-elements.[18-26] These images are obtained using the technique of absorption contrast.

There are two excellent reviews of micro X-ray CT using SR.[27-28] The first

Tohoru Takeda MD PhD, Assistant Professor, Institute of Clinical Medicine, University of Tsukuba, 1–1–1 Tennodai, Tsukuba-shi, Ibaraki 305–8575 Japan

Yuji Itai MD PhD, Professor, Institute of Clinical Medicine, University of Tsukuba, 1-1-1 Tennodai, Tsukuba-shi, Ibaraki 305-8575 Japan

describes the detailed physics of transmission of micro X-ray CT, and the paper by Bonse and Busch describes transmission micro X-ray CT and phase-contrast micro X-ray CT.

In this chapter, we will first discuss the properties of synchrotron radiation that make it suitable for micro X-ray CT followed by a review of the various kinds of X-ray CT with SR, such as transmission X-ray, fluorescent X-ray and phase-contrast X-ray.

THE PROPERTIES OF SYNCHROTRON RADIATION FOR X-RAY CT IMAGING

For a relativistic electron forced by a magnetic field, the radiation pattern has to be transformed using a Lorentz transformation into the laboratory system.[29] This produces radiation (synchrotron radiation) within a small cone only, which has an opening angle of $\theta \sim 1/\gamma$, as illustrated in Fig. 6.1:

$$\gamma = E/E_o$$

where E is the energy of the electron in units of its rest energy (E_0 which = 0.511 MeV).

Synchrotron radiation has several advantageous properties that make it suitable for use in X-ray CT. These are listed below.

1. High photon flux density to enhance the signal intensity (Fig. 6.2).
2. Natural forwarding of collimation for focusing the incident X-rays.
3. Broad energy spectrum that allows tunability of beam energy to excite the relevant atoms.
4. Linear polarization.

The merits of SR for use in the X-ray CT are listed in Table 6.1.

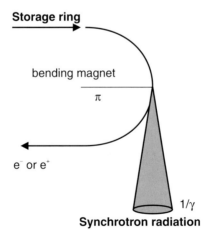

Fig. 6.1 Generation of synchrotron radiation.

Table 6.1 Advantages of synchrotron radiation for X-ray CT

Advantages for X-ray CT	Relevant property of synchrotron radiation
Imaging of specific elements (optimum absorption contrast and minimal radiation damage)	Broad energy spectrum (selection of proper X-ray energy) High flux density
High spatial resolution	Natural forwarding of collimation High flux density
Absolute CT number	Absence of beam hardening effects (monochromatic X-ray) Highly natural collimation (reduction of scattering radiation) High flux density
High speed imaging	High flux density

CT = computed tomography

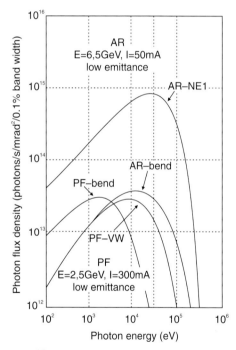

AR = accumulation ring
NEI = beam line number of multiple wiggler
PF = Photon Factory, High Energy Accelerator Research Organisation, Tsukuba, Japan
VW = vertical wiggler

Fig. 6.2 The relationship between the photon flux and energy in synchrotron radiation.

THE FORMATION OF MONOCHROMATIC X-RAYS

For X-ray CT imaging, the use of monochromatic X-rays has significant merits, such as high contrast, the ability to perform quantitative analyses due to the highly sensitive detection of specific elements and non-beam hardening. The X-ray energy can be tuned optimally by Bragg reflection or Laue diffraction.

In Bragg reflection, an X-ray quantum falling upon a semi-infinite slab of a

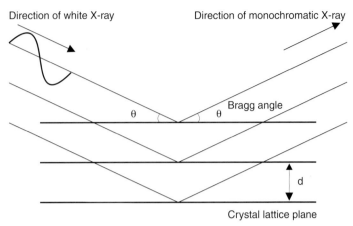

Fig. 6.3 The energy selection by Bragg reflection.

perfect single crystal may be coherently reflected from the crystal if the wavelength and angle with respect to the crystal lattice satisfy the familiar Bragg equation (Fig. 6.3):

$\lambda = 2d \sin \theta$

where d is the lattice spacing and θ is the angle of the quantum with respect to the lattice planes.

CONTRAST FORMATION OF X-RAY IMAGING

Image contrast originates from the modulation of the probing radiation. The interaction between the X-ray and the object simultaneously produces a fluorescent X-ray, a scattering X-ray (with both Compton and Thomson scattering) and a refraction (phase-shift) X-ray (Fig. 6.4). The refraction X-ray has a very small angle difference of less than $10^{-4} - 10^{-6}$, compared to the transmission X-ray. After several interactions between the X-ray and the object, the transmitted X-ray is obtained. Currently in X-ray imaging, the contrast X-ray image is generated by

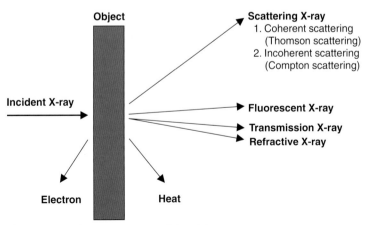

Fig. 6.4 The interaction between X-rays and the object.

Table 6.2 Various types of X-ray computed tomography with synchrotron radiation

a)	Transmission types
	High spatial resolution CT
	High contrast resolution CT
	Three-dimensional CT by fluorescent X-ray source
b)	Fluorescent scanning X-ray CT
c)	Scattering CT (Compton & Thomson)
d)	Phase contrast X-ray CT

the transmitted X-ray, which is mainly produced as a result of the photoelectric effect and the Compton (incoherent) scattering effect. Image contrast arises from a variation of μ within the sample material:

$$N = N_0 \exp(-\Sigma\mu_s d_s)$$

where N and N_0 are the photon number of transmission X-rays and incident X-rays, respectively. $\Sigma\mu$ is the integrated attenuation coefficient along the path of the X-rays travelling through the sample.

Based on the above physical properties, a monochromatic synchrotron X-ray with high flux would enable the development of various types of CT (Table 6.2).

X-RAY CT WITH SR

TRANSMISSION X-RAY CT

HIGH SPATIAL RESOLUTION X-RAY CT

High spatial resolution X-ray CT with SR has been used in both industrial and in material science investigations.[30-36] Since absorption of X-rays by a biological object (soft tissue) is very small, high spatial resolution X-ray CT is better suited for imaging relatively high density objects or organs, such as bone structures and teeth. This method provides excellent contrast and has a spatial resolution capacity ranging from 2–100 μm.

High spatial resolution X-ray CT system

The high spatial resolution X-ray CT system consists of a slit array, a rotating table component, a double-crystal monochromator and an X-ray detector (Fig. 6.5). The double-crystal arrangement is used to obtain both monochromatic x-ray beam and object magnification (asymmetric reflection), and to decrease the contamination arising from the higher-order harmonics of the Bragg reflection. The X-ray energy is adjustable from 20–100 keV. Image magnification can also range from 25 times (corresponding spatial resolution = 2 μm) to 0.5 times by combining an asymmetric Bragg reflection of the X-ray on to the second mirror using a light lens system.[37]

Experimental parameters and imaging of a rat skull

In an experiment to image the skull of a live rat, the size of the object was larger than that of the detector, so a symmetric reflection crystal was used as the second crystal. The charged coupled device (CCD) array element size was 22 μm × 22 μm with a dynamic range of 10^5, and was cooled with liquid nitrogen to reduce the dark current. The output signal was digitized using a 16-bit analog-to-digital converter. The CT image was reconstructed using a filtered back-projection

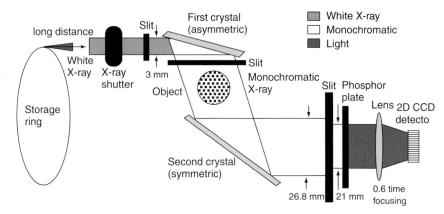

Fig. 6.5 Schematic diagram of the high spatial resolution X-ray CT system. 2D, two-dimensional.

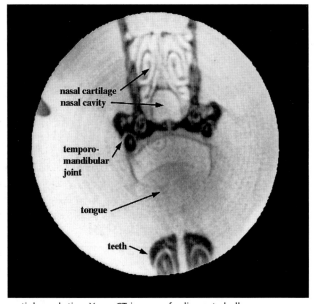

Fig. 6.6 High spatial resolution X-ray CT image of a live rat skull.

method. The incident monochromatic X-ray flux ahead of sensor was about 10^7 photons mm^{-2} s^{-1}.

The image of a live rat skull was obtained using a slice thickness of 36-μm and 33.2-keV X-ray energy.[9] The nasal cartilage, skull and teeth of the live rat were clearly demonstrated (Fig. 6.6).

Currently, the main research fields that use this system are those involved in imaging three-dimensional bony structures to evaluate osteoporosis and bone remodelling.[10-14]

HIGH CONTRAST RESOLUTION X-RAY CT

A highly sensitive X-ray CT with SR was constructed to generate a map of the distribution of low and intermediate Z-elements (P, S, Cl, K, Ca and Fe) using a linear array detector composed of high purity germanium or a $CdWO_4$ scintillator/diode,[15–17] and has been developed to reveal the distribution of high Z-elements (I and Gd)[18–24] for neurological diagnosis. Recently an excellent in vivo image of rat brain tumours has been obtained.[25]

Minimal detectability of contrast elements
In the ideal state (without scatter radiation), the minimal detectability of the contrast element can be calculated from the noise due to the photon counting statistics in CT.[38] The signal-to-noise (S/N) ratio (σ^2/μ^2) is defined by the equation:

$$\frac{\sigma^2}{\mu^2} = \frac{\pi^2 \int_{-00}^{00} k^2 \,|W(k)|^2 dk}{m^2\mu^2} \sum_{j=1}^{m} \left(\frac{1}{N_j}\right)$$

where μ is the true value of the attenuation coefficient and σ^2 is the variance of the measured attenuation at a particular point. m is the number of projections, N_j is the photon flux density (photons/mm^2) of the unscattered photons that have passed through the element of interest and are detected in the jth projection, and W(k) is the window function of the corrective filter for the reconstruction.

Using the above equation, the relationship between the minimal detectability of iodine and the photon flux density can be calculated (Fig. 6.7).[22] The theoretical minimal detectable concentration of iodine is 35.3 μg/ml; μ = 177.0 (cm^{-1}) (above K-edge energy), m = 180, N_j = 1.0 × 10^6 photons/mm^2/projection (7.0 × 10^7 photons/mm^2/s × 0.04 × exp(–0.33 × 3)), at 0.2-mm spatial resolution and 1-mm slice thickness.

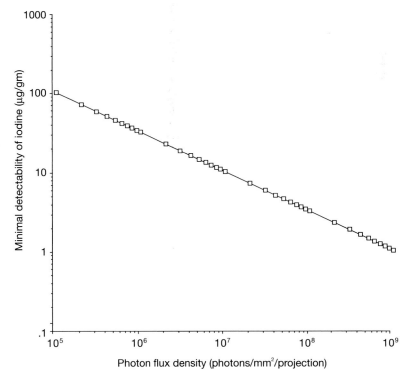

Fig. 6.7 Minimal detectability of an iodine contrast element. —□—, 0.2 mm × 0.2 mm × 1.0 mm.

FLUORESCENT X-RAY CT

Fluorescent X-ray analysis is commonly used to detect very low concentrations of elements (in the order of picograms),[39] but these measurements require thin specimen slices that are scanned perpendicular to the surface. Although the focusing X-ray beam size becomes only a few μm, still the excited X-ray energy is less than 28 keV (mostly less than 20 keV) because the main targets are low and intermediate Z-elements (Ca, Fe, Cu and Zn).

For non-destructive fluorescent X-ray imaging, the fluorescent tomogram and fluorescent X-ray computed tomography (FXCT) have been developed. A fluorescent tomogram device using X-ray tubes has shown the presence of 5 mg iodine in a volume of 2.5×2.6×2.5 mm³,[40] and micro-tomography with SR has been used to show the presence of iron in the head of a bee.[41] Fluorescent X-ray tomography with SR detected about 200 ng iodine in a volume of 4 mm³.[42–45] The detectability of the iodine content was improved by the reduction of Compton scattering overlapping the fluorescent K shell α line due to the highest linear polarization of the synchrotron X-rays.

FXCT is being developed for the detection of non-radioactive contrast materials (high Z-elements) in living specimens, in a similar way to the images obtained using radionuclide examinations with single photon emission computed tomography (SPECT) scans.[46] A FXCT image was obtained using 37 keV monochromatic synchrotron X-rays and a parallel collimator. This system could detect about 60 ng iodine in a volume of 1 mm³.[47] FXCT was used to depict the two-dimensional distribution of iodine within the thyroid gland,[48–50] and to depict the distribution of iodine solution and xenon gas within a phantom.[51,52] There are some possibilities for imaging the high Z-elements of pathological specimens, such as platinum-containing anti-cancer drugs within a tumour,[45] and the intermediate Z-elements such as zinc and copper within a renal tumour (12.3 ± 5.05 μg/g and 0.99 ± 0.50 μg/g, respectively).[53]

The principles and properties of fluorescent X-rays, the FXCT system and their biomedical application are described below.

FLUORESCENT X-RAYS

Fluorescent X-rays are induced by the transition of atomic-orbital electrons from high- to low-energy states after the excitation of the inner orbital electrons by primary X-ray photons (Fig. 6.8).[39] The emitted X-ray energy spectrum is characteristic of the excited element (Table 6.3), and the intensity of the spectral lines is proportional to the amount of that element contained in the sample from:

$$I_{fluorescent} = \alpha C I_0 \exp\{-(\Sigma\mu_I d_I + \Sigma\mu_F d_F)\}$$

where I_0 is the incident monochromatic X-ray flux ahead of the specimens, μ_I and d_I are the linear attenuation of the incident monochromatic X-ray and the absorption length, respectively. α is the excitation ratio of fluorescent X-rays and C is the concentration of the target element.

For the fluorescent X-ray analysis, the linear polarization of SR in the plane of the electron storage ring is the most important property for detecting very low concentrations of specific elements because of the significant reduction of spectral background radiation originating from Compton scattering. The polarization

Table 6.3 Excitation energy and fluorescent X-ray energy of intermediate and high Z-elements

	Excitation energy	$K_{\alpha 1}$	$K_{\alpha 2}$	$K_{\beta 1}$	$K_{\beta 2}$
Intermediate Z-elements					
Calcium (20)	>4.039	3.69	3.68	4.01	
Iron (26)	>7.111	6.40	6.39	7.05	
Copper (29)	>8.981	8.04	8.02	8.90	
Zinc (30)	>9.661	9.63	8.61	9.57	
Bromine (35)	>13.474	11.92	11.87	13.29	
High Z-elements					
Iodine (53)	>33.170	28.61	28.32	32.3	33.0
Xenon (54)	>34.566	29.78	29.46	33.6	34.4
Gadolinium (64)	>50.239	43.0	42.31	48.7	50.0
Ytterbium (70)	>61.332	52.39	51.35	59.3	61.0
Platinum (78)	>78.395	66.83	65.12	75.7	77.8
Lead (82)	>88.005	74.96	72.80	84.93	

The number in parenthesis after each element name is the atomic number.

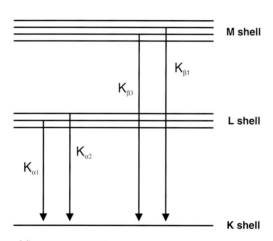

Fig. 6.8 Generation of fluorescent X-rays.

allows an almost complete suppression of the Compton scattering by positioning the detector at a 90-degree angle to the beam in the plane of polarization (Fig. 6.9). As a result, the minimal detectable limit obtained with SR is less than 1 picogram, i.e. $10^3 - 10^4$-fold less than that obtained with a conventional X-ray tube beam.

FLUORESCENT X-RAY CT SYSTEM

The FXCT system consists of a silicon (111) double crystal monochromator, an X-ray shutter, an X-ray slit system, a scanning table for the target organ and an X-ray detector for both fluorescent and transmission X-rays (Fig. 6.10). The white X-ray beam is monochromatized using silicon (111) double crystal in the Bragg–Bragg configuration. This monochromatized X-ray is collimated into a pencil beam using a thin tantalum slit. The fluorescent X-ray, which is being emitted isotropically along the line of the incident X-ray beam, is detected in a highly purified germanium (HPGe) detector operating in a photon-counting mode. The HPGe detector is positioned perpendicular to the incident

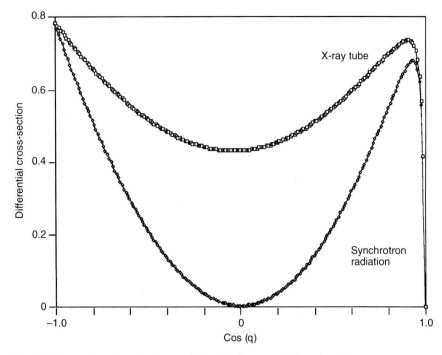

Fig. 6.9 The merits of synchrotron radiation for fluorescent X-ray imaging.

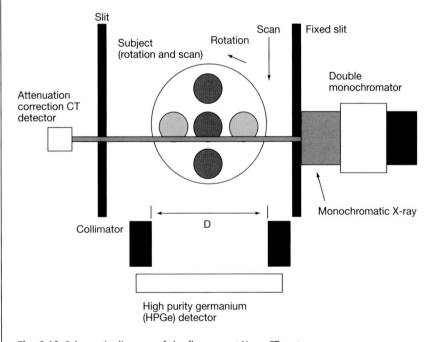

Fig. 6.10 Schematic diagram of the fluorescent X-ray CT system.

monochromatic X-ray beam, and was collimated by a parallel beam to reduce the amount of stray radiation reaching the detector.

Projection data are acquired at constant angular steps using a translation–rotation motion of the subject over 180°. The subject's motion is facilitated by a stepping motor.

The counts under the characteristic fluorescent K_α X-ray spectral lines at each projection are used to generate the CT projection. The transmission X-ray beam is measured by the X-ray CCD detector together with the fluorescent X-rays, and the attenuation corrections of the incident beam and the emitted fluorescent X-rays are applied to each projection using transmission X-ray CT image data.

FXCT images are reconstructed using the least-squares method, taking the singular value of decomposition with simultaneous correcting of the beam obtained using the X-ray absorption method.[54]

EXPERIMENTAL PARAMETER AND OBJECTS

An experiment was carried out at the bending magnet beam of line the Tristan accumulation ring (6.5 GeV, 10–30 mA) in Tsukuba, Japan. The energy of the monochromatic X-ray beam was adjusted to 37.0 keV. Using an ion chamber, the measured photon flux rate in front of the object was approximately 7×10^7 photons/mm²/s at a beam current of 30 mA.

The monochromatic X-ray beam was collimated into a 1×1 mm² beam (horizontal and vertical, respectively) using an X-ray slit. In the detecting portion, excited fluorescent X-rays were also collimated to 1×30 mm² $\times 100$ mm length. The distance between the HPGe detector and the specimen was 200 mm. The data acquisition time was 20 s at each scanning point. Projection data were acquired at 3° steps using a translation–rotation motion of the subject over 180°.

The transmission X-ray beam was measured using a water-cooled X-ray CCD detector that had a 22.5-μm spatial resolution with 16-bit analogue to digital (A/D) converter. The data acquisition time was 0.2 s at each scanning point. Transmission X-ray CT images were reconstructed using a filtered back projection method.

The objects were a 20 mm diameter fixed in formalin human thyroid gland and a 30 mm diameter two-element imaging phantom containing a 2 mg iodine solution and 30% xenon gas.

FLUORESCENT X-RAY CT IMAGES

The K_α and $K_{\beta1}$ fluorescent X-ray lines of iodine within the thyroid gland, Compton scattering and Thomson scattering are shown in Fig. 6.11. The distribution of iodine within the thyroid gland from a patient with hyperthyroidism was not uniform (Fig. 6.12) in spite of a homogeneously high uptake, as demonstrated by an I-123 scintigram. Pathological studies could not show a heterogeneous distribution of iodine. The iodine content within the thyroid gland and the thyroid cancer lesion can be evaluated quantitatively. The iodine content of the thyroid cancer lesion was very small, it was less than 0.2 mg/g.[48,50]

A linear correlation was observed between the iodine concentration and the fluorescent X-ray counts from the phantom sample, and the minimum detectable concentration of iodine solution was estimated at 30 ng in a volume of 1 mm³. In

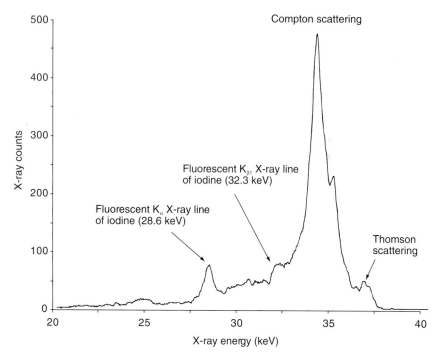

Fig. 6.11 The spectrum obtained using fluorescent X-ray CT with a human thyroid gland sample.

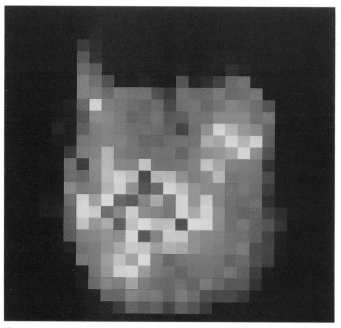

Fig. 6.12 Fluorescent X-ray CT image of a thyroid gland with hyperthyroidism.

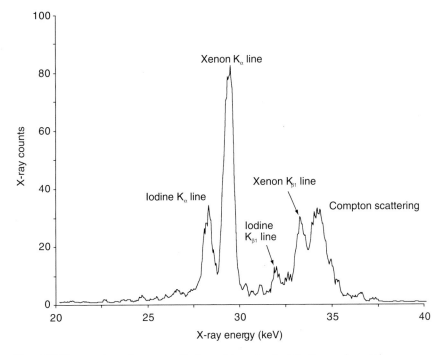

Fig. 6.13 The spectrum from a multi-element imaging test (iodine and xenon).

the multi-element imaging test, the K_α and $K_{\beta 1}$ fluorescent X-ray lines of iodine and xenon were clearly differentiated (Fig. 6.13).

Currently, high spatial resolution types of FXCT systems are being developed to obtain spatial resolutions of less than 200 μm and a data acquisition time of less than 5 s at each scanning point.

FXCT can be used to detect high Z-elements at low concentrations and to clearly delineate their distribution quantitatively. Although the intermediate Z-elements could also possibly be imaged using FXCT, the observation area must be a vacuum to reduce the absorption of the fluorescent X-rays by air.

PHASE-CONTRAST X-RAY CT

At present, clinical X-ray images simply describe the distribution of the linear attenuation coefficient. However, the discrimination between tumour lesions and normal tissues is difficult because the difference in the linear attenuation coefficient of biological objects is very small.

Recently, several imaging techniques for detecting the hard X-ray phase shift are being developed because the phase-shift cross-section is much larger than the absorption cross-section and hence a high sensitivity to biological objects is expected. These techniques include an interferometric method[18, 55–57] using a crystal X-ray interferometer,[58] a Schlieren-like method using crystal diffraction,[59–63] a holography-like method,[64–67] and others.[68–70] The Schlieren-like method using crystal diffraction and the holography-like method are adequate for imaging an object with significant density difference between the soft tissue, calcification, fat and air. Among these methods, an interferometric method using a crystal X-ray interferometer is considered to be the most sensitive method.

Using an X-ray interferometer, phase-contrast X-ray radiography with SR revealed the cerebellar structures of a rat[56] and human metastatic tumour lesions[57] without the contrast element. Phase-contrast X-ray CT[71] also demonstrated rabbit cancer lesions,[72-74] the rat cerebrum[27, 75] and human cancer lesions.[76-80]

The principles of phase-contrast X-ray imaging, the phase-contrast X-ray CT system, imaging of biological objects and future application are described below.

PRINCIPLES OF PHASE-CONTRAST X-RAY IMAGING

The formal principles underlying phase-contrast imaging are presented here. The refraction index n is given by:

$$n = 1 - \delta - i\beta$$

where

$$\delta = r_e \lambda^2 / 2\pi \Sigma N_1 (Z_1 + f^r_1)$$

and

$$\beta = r_e \lambda^2 / 2\pi \Sigma \ (N_1 f^i_1)$$

Here N_1 is the number of atoms per unit volume for element 1; Z_1 is the atomic number; f^r_1 and f^i_1 are the real and imaginary parts of the anomalous atomic scattering factor at the wavelength λ, respectively; $r_e (= e^2 / mc^2)$ is the classical electron radius; c, e and m are fundamental constants. $N_1 Z_1$ is proportional to the density of element 1 inside the sample. Only δ affects the phase-shift, and the value of p for element 1 in the object is given[56] by:

$$p_1 = r_e \lambda (Z_1 + f^r_1).$$

The ratio between the equivalent X-ray phase-shift cross-section p and the total absorption cross-section μ_a is calculated as p/μ_a at an X-ray energy of 13.5 keV as a function of the atomic number Z (Fig. 6.14). The values of μ_a and f^r_1 were obtained from the data in the atomic table edited by Sasaki.[81]

The value of p is more than 1000 times larger than μ_a for light elements. Furthermore, the value of p is larger than μ_a for heavy elements. Thus, for biological objects, consisting of hydrogen, carbon, nitrogen and oxygen atoms, the signal-to-noise ratio for the image of a single atom is expected to be larger by more than 1000 times compared to that obtained with the conventional radiography method using contrast absorption.

PHASE-CONTRAST X-RAY CT SYSTEM

The phase-contrast X-ray CT apparatus consists of an asymmetric silicon crystal (220), a triple Laue-case X-ray interferometer (silicon (220)),[72] and an X-ray detector system (Fig. 6.15). The X-ray interferometer is made from a highly perfect single-crystal block by cutting two wide grooves in the block. This interferometer has three parallel X-ray half mirrors called the beam splitter, the mirror and the analyzer. By means of Laue diffraction on the beam splitter, the incident x-ray beam is divided into two coherent beams. These beams are spatially separated

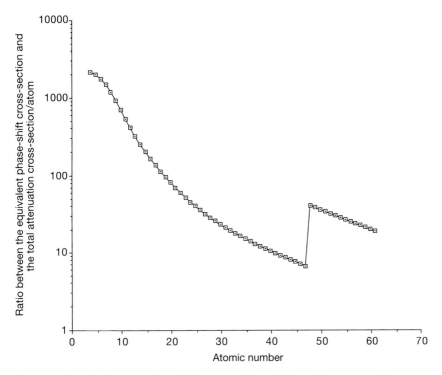

Fig. 6.14 The ratio between phase-shift cross-section and absorption cross-section.
—□—, 13.5 keV e-ray energy.

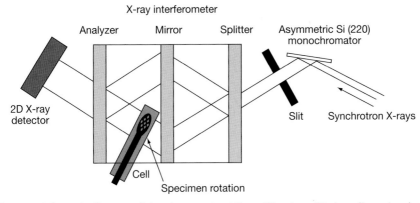

Fig. 6.15 Schematic diagram of the phase-contrast X-ray CT system. 2D, two-dimensional.

before they reach the mirror, where they are again reflected by Laue diffraction. Two converged beams from the four beams generated by the mirror, are overlapped on the entrance surface of the analyzer. The analyzer combines these beams and an X-ray interference pattern appears in the outgoing beams from the back surface of the analyzer.

EXPERIMENTAL PARAMETERS AND OBJECTS

An experiment was performed at a vertical wiggler beam line of the Photon Factory in Tsukuba, Japan. The X-ray energy was set at 17.7 keV, and the X-ray flux in front of the sample was estimated to be about 5×10^5 photons/mm^2/s. The typical beam current of the storage ring was 300 mA with 2.5 GeV.

A specimen was placed in a cell filled with water. The cell was inserted into the beams path between the mirror and the analyzer of the interferometer as shown in Fig. 6.15. Since the position of the beam was fixed, the specimens were rotated within the cell. The field of view was limited to 5 mm × 5 mm, so a column specimen smaller than 5-mm was cut from pathological tissues. The beam exposure time was 60 s/projection and the number of projections was 200 over 180°. Phase-contrast X-ray CT images were reconstructed with a voxel size of 12 μm, however the current spatial resolution was about 30 μm.[72] The image reconstruction methods have been previously described.[71]

The specimens, fixed in formalin, consisted of a case of metastatic colon cancer in the liver and a case of normal breast tissue.

PHASE-CONTRAST X-RAY CT IMAGING

Phase-contrast X-ray CT images mapped the difference (dδ) between the refractive index of the tissue in the sample and the refractive index of water at 17.7 keV X-ray energy. Phase-contrast X-ray CT clearly revealed various structures within the human pathological specimens such as cancer cells, necrotic tissue and capsulated fibrosis in the case of metastatic colon carcinoma in the liver (Fig. 6.16), and fibrotic tissue in normal breast (Fig. 6.17) at slice thickness of 12 μm. Images produced by phase-contrast X-ray CT were similar to 20-times magnified optical microscopic images. However, the very fine morphological

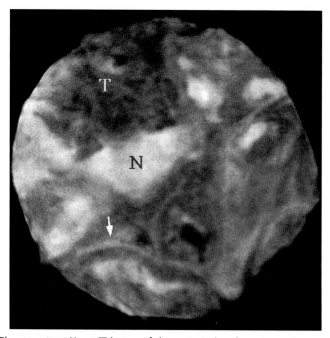

Fig. 6.16 Phase-contrast X-ray CT image of the metastatic colon cancer. Cancer cells are shown as mosaic-like low density structures (T, tumour), whereas necrosis is shown as significantly high density areas with complex structures (N, necrosis). Fibrotic capsule is shown as a thin high density linear band (arrow).

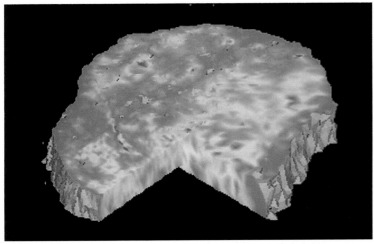

Fig. 6.17 Three dimensional phase-contrast X-ray CT image of the normal breast. Dense fibrotic tissues and the surrounding rough fibrotic tissues are shown as a three-dimensional network, from yellow to orange colour and the green area, respectively. Adipose tissues are demonstrated as blue spot lesions.

structures of specimens were not clearly imaged by this phase-contrast X-ray CT because of the 30 μm spatial resolution.

Cancer cells had low dδ value compared to normal liver tissue, which is in agreement with results obtained from phase-contrast X-ray CT images of virus induced rabbit papilloma (VX-2) cancer of rabbits[72-74] and various human cancers.[76-80] Necrotic tissue has a high dδ value compared to normal liver tissue. Fibrotic capsules had a relatively high dδ value in these pathological specimens, but a previous study on breast tumours has revealed that the dδ of fibrosis depends on the roughness of the fibrotic tissue.[77]

In addition, we are now trying to image the vessel structures without using contrast elements such as iodine.[82]

PRESENT LIMITATIONS AND FUTURE PLANS

For medical applications, the most important problem is establishing a method to expand the field of view. In the present phase-contrast X-ray imaging system, the view size of the object is limited to 5 mm × 5 mm due to the small size of the X-ray interferometer that is manufactured using a 7.62-cm diameter silicon ingot. To increase the field of view to image larger samples, larger monolithic X-ray inter-ferometers [83] and separated-type interferometers[84-87] are now being developed. At present, the largest available diameter of the silicon ingot is 10-cm, therefore an image of 25 mm × 25 mm is possible. Using this interferometer, phase-contrast CT images and in vivo phase-contrast projection images are being obtained. A sepa-rated-type interferometer is currently being developed to obtain a field of view of about 100 mm × 100 mm.[87] Using this separated-type interferometer, we are plan-ning to perform phase-contrast X-ray mammography in vivo.

In addition, the current spatial resolution of our system is limited to about 30 μm due to the diffraction phenomenon within the crystal wafers.[88] This aspect can be improved by manufacturing a thin wafer. For example, it is expected that a spatial resolution of less than 10 μm could be achieved by using a 100-μm thick wafer (analyzer).

KEY POINTS

1. New types of micro X-ray CT such as transmission X-ray and phase-contrast X-ray have been described.
2. In particular, the phase-contrast X-ray CT, which generates contrast from differences in refractive indices, has great potential for revealing the micro-structures inside soft tissues without the contrast element because of its high sensitivity for biological objects.
3. FXCT is now being developed to image the specific element distribution at a spatial resolution of less than 0.2 mm.

ACKNOWLEDGEMENT

We would like to thank the following: Takao Akatsuka PhD, Tetsuya Yuasa PhD, Jin Wu MD, PhD, Akira Uchida PhD, Quanwen Yu PhD, Tsutomu Zeniya MS, Toshikazu Maeda MS, Masahiro Akiba MS, Masahiro Kazama MS, Yuki Hoshino MS, Naoto Kusaka MS and Yasuhiro Hasegawa Mr, for their help with FXCT and transmission X-ray CT experiments; Kazuo Hayashi MS, Yasuaki Nagata MS and Hironao Yamaji MS for their help with high spatial resolution X-ray CT; Atsushi Momose PhD for his help with phase-contrast X-ray imaging; Kazuyuki Hyodo PhD and Keiichi Hirano PhD for their technical support of experiments in the Photon Factory; Tristan AR Ring, Ei Ueno MD, PhD, Toru Yashiro MD, PhD, Seiji Haraoka MD, PhD and Teruo Watanabe MD, PhD for the preparation of pathological tissues.

This research was partially supported by a Grant-in-aid for Scientific Research (No.08407024, No.10557084) and Developmental Science Research grant (No.06507002) from the Japanese Ministry of Education, Science and Culture. This study was performed under the auspices of the National Laboratory for High Energy Physics (Proposal Nos 95G289, 95G349, 97G163, 97G164, 99G124, 99S2–002).

REFERENCES

1. Hounsfield GN. Computerized transverse axial scanning (tomography): Part 1. Description of system. Br J Radiol 1973; 46: 1016–1022
2. Meyer JS, Hayman LA, Yamamoto M, Sakai F, Nakajima S. Local cerebral blood flow measured by CT after stable xenon inhalation. Am J Roentgen 1980; 135: 239–251
3. Winkler SS, Sackett JF, Holden JE et al. Xenon inhalation as an adjunct to computerized tomography of the brain: preliminary study. Invest Radiol 1977; 12: 15–18
4. Grodzins L. Optimum energies for X-ray transmission tomography of small samples. Application of synchrotron radiation to computed tomography I. Nucl Instr Meth 1983; 206: 541–545
5. Grodzins L. Critical absorption tomography of small samples. Proposed application of synchrotron radiation to computed tomography II. Nucl Instr Meth 1983; 206: 547–552
6. Thompson AC, Llacer J, Campbell Finman L, Hughes EB, Wilson S, Zeman HD. Computed tomography using synchrotron radiation. Nucl Instr Meth 1984; 222: 319–323

7. Borodin Y, Dementyev EN, Dragun GN et al. Scanning X-ray difference microscopy and microtomography using synchrotron radiation of the storage ring VEPP-4. Nucl Instr Meth 1986; A 246: 649–654
8. Engelke K, Lohmann M. A system for dual energy microtomography of bones. Nucl Instr Meth Phys Res 1989; A 274: 380–389
9. Takeda T, Itai Y, Hayashi K, Nagata Y, Yamaji H, Hyodo K. High spatial resolution CT with a synchrotron radiation system. J Comp Assist Tomogr 1994; 18: 98–101
10. Bonse U, Busch F, Gunnewig O et al. 3D computed X-ray tomography of human cancellous bone at 8 um spatial and 10^{-4} energy resolution. Bone Mineral 1994; 25: 25–38
11. Hildebrand T, Laib A, Ulrich D, Kohlbrenner A, Ruegsegger P. Bone structure as revealed by microtomography. In: Proceedings from Developments in X-ray Tomography. Society of Photo-optical Instrument Engineers. (SPIE) 1997; 3149: 34–43
12. Engelke K, UmgieBer G, Prevhal S, Kalender W. Three-dimensional analysis of trabecular bone structure: the need for spongiosa standard models. In: Proceedings from Developments in X-ray Tomography. SPIE 1997; 3149: 53–61
13. Kinney JH, Haupt DL, Ladd AJC. Applications of synchrotron microtomography in osteoporosis research. In: Proceedings from Developments in X-ray Tomography. SPIE 1997; 3149: 64–68
14. Muller R, Wilson CH. Biomechanical competence of micro structural bone in the progress of adaptive bone remodeling. In: Proceedings from Developments in X-ray Tomography. SPIE 1997; 3149: 69–81
15. Dilmanian FA, Garrett RF, Thomlinson WC et al. Computed tomography with monochromatic X rays from the National Synchrotron Light Source. Nucl Instr Meth 1991; B56/57: 1208–1213
16. Nachaliel E, Dilmanian FA, Garrett RF et al. Monochromatic computed tomography of the human brain using synchrotron X-rays: technical feasibility. Nucl Instr Meth 1992; A319: 305–310
17. Dilmanian FA. Computed tomography with monochromatic X-rays. Am J Physiol Imaging 1992; 3/4: 175–193
18. Dilmanian FA, Wu XY, Parsons EC et al. Single- and dual-energy CT with monochromatic synchrotron X-rays. Phys Med Biol 1997; 42: 371–387
19. Takeda T, Akatsuka T, Hyodo K et al. Synchrotron radiation x-ray computed tomography to detect tracer material. Med Imaging Technol 1992; 10: 299–300
20. Itai Y, Takeda T, Akatsuka T et al. High contrast computed tomography with synchrotron radiation. Rev Sci Instrum 1995; 66: 1385–1387
21. Zeniya T, Takeda T, Hyodo K et al. Detectability of tracer materials in synchrotron radiation X-ray computed tomography: Preliminary experiments using a prototype system with imaging plate as a detector. Med Imaging Technol 1997; 15: 121–137 (Abstract in English)
22. Kazama M, Takeda T, Akiba M et al. Performance study of monochromatic synchrotron X-ray computed tomography using a linear array detector. Med Imaging Technol 1997; 15: 615–624
23. Takeda T, Kazama M, Zeniya T et al. Development of a monochromatic X-ray computed tomography with synchrotron radiation for functional imaging. In: Ando M, Uyama C (Eds) Medical Applications of Synchrotron Radiation. Tokyo: Springer-Verlag, 1998; 103–110
24. Charvet AM, Latizien C, Esteve F et al. Synchrotron radiation computed tomography applied to the brain: phantom studies at the ESRF medical beamline. In: Ando M, Uyama C (Eds) Medical Applications of Synchrotron Radiation. Tokyo: Springer-Verlag, 1998; 95–98
25. Le Duc G, Charvet AM, Elleaume H, Esteve F, Collomb A, Lebas JF. In vivo imaging of brain tumors in rats by K-edge SRCT using iodine and gadolinium contrast agents. Synchr Rad News 1999; 12: 28–33
26. Saito T, Kudo H, Takeda T et al. Three-dimensional monochromatic X-ray computed tomography using synchrotron radiation. Optical Engin 1998; 37: 2258–2268
27. Graeff W, Engelke K. Microradiography and microtomography. In: Ebashi S, Koch M, Rubenstein E (Eds), Handbook on Synchrotron Radiation, vol 4. Amsterdam: North-Holland, 1991; 361–405

28. Bonse U, Busch F. X-ray computed microtomography (μCT) using synchrotron radiation (SR). Prog Biophy Mol Biol 1996; 65: 133–169

29. Brefeld W, Gurtler P. Synchrotron radiation sources. In: Ebashi S, Koch M, Rubenstein E (Eds) Handbook on Synchrotron Radiation, vol. 4. Amsterdam: North-Holland, 1991; 269–296

30. Flannery BP, Deckman HW, Roberge WG, D'Amico KL. Three-dimensional X-ray micro-tomography. Science 1987; 237: 1439–1444

31. Suzuki Y, Usami K, Sakamoto K et al. X-ray computerized tomography using monochromated synchrotron radiation. Jpn J Appl Phys 1988; 27: L461–464

32. Hirano T, Usami K, Sakamoto K. High resolution monochromatic tomography with X-ray sensing pickup tube. Rev Sci Instrum 1989; 60: 2482–2485

33. Kinney JH, Johnson QC, Nichols MC et al. X-ray microtomography on beamline X at SSRL. Rev Sci Instrum 1989; 60: 2471–2474

34. Nubhardt R, Bonse U, Busch F, Kinney JH, Saroyan RA, Nichols MC. Microtomography: a tool for nondestructive study of materials. Synchr Rad News 1991; 4: 21–23

35. D'Amico KL, Dunsmuir JH, Ferguson SR, Flannery BP, Deckman HW. The Exxon micro-tomography beam line at the National Synchrotron Light Source. Rev Sci Instrum 1992; 63: 574–577

36. Nagata Y, Yamaji H, Hayashi K et al. High energy high resolution monochromatic X-ray computed tomography using the Photon Factory vertical wiggler beamline. Rev Sci Instrum 1992; 63: 615–618

37. Nagata Y, Yamaji H, Hayashi K et al. High energy, high resolution monochromatic X-ray computed tomography system. Res Nondestr Eval 1992; 4: 55–78

38. Chesler DA, Riederer SJ, Pelc NJ. Noise due to photon counting statistics in computed x-ray tomography. J Comput Assist Tomogr 1977; 1: 64–74

39. Iida A, Gohshi Y. Trace element analysis by X-ray fluorescence. In: Ebashi S, Koch M, Rubenstein E (Eds) Handbook on Synchrotron Radiation, vol. 4. Amsterdam: North-Holland, 1991; 307–348

40. Cesareo R, Mascarenhas S. A new tomographic device based on the detection of fluorescent X-rays. Nucl Instr Meth 1989; A277: 669–672

41. Boisseau P, Grodzins L. Fluorescence tomography using synchrotron radiation. Hyperfine Interact 1987; 33: 283–292

42. Takeda T, Ito K, Kishi K et al. Preliminary experiment of the fluorescent X-ray computed tomography with synchrotron radiation. Med Imaging Technol 1994; 12: 537–538

43. Takeda T. Fluorescent CT with monochromatic X-rays from Tristan accumulation ring. (Abstract in poster CB2) The 13th International Accelerator Conference, Denton, Texas, 7–10 Nov 1994

44. Takeda T, Maeda T, Yuasa T et al. Fluorescent scanning X-ray tomography with synchrotron radiation. Rev Sci Instr 1995; 66: 1471–1473

45. Takeda T, Maeda T, Yuasa T et al. Fluorescent scanning X-ray tomographic image with monochromatic synchrotron X-ray. Med Imaging Technol 1996; 14: 183–194

46. Takeda T, Akiba M, Yuasa T, Kazama M, Hoshino Y, Hyodo K, Dilmanian FA, Akatsuka T, Itai Y. Fluorescent x-ray computed tomography with synchrotron radiation using fan collimator. SPIE 1996; 2708: 685–695

47. Takeda T, Yuasa T, Hosino A, Akiba M, Uchida A, Kazama M, Hyodo K, Dilmanian FA, Akatsuka T, Itai Y. Fluorescent x-ray computed tomography to visualize specific material distribution. SPIE 1997; 3149: 160–172

48. Takeda T, Doi T, Ohtsuka S, Sugishita Y, Saito T, ItaiY, Momose A, Umetani K, Hyodo K, Ando M, Toyofuku F, Tokumori K, Uyama C, Yu Q, Yuasa T, Akatsuka T. Recent topics of synchrotron x-ray imaging for medical research in Japan. Program abstract p60, 6th International Conference on Biophysics & Synchrotron Radiation (Argonne, USA) August 4–8, 1998

49. Rust GF, Weigelt J. X-ray fluorescent computer tomography with synchrotron radiation. IEEE TransNuclSci 1998; 45: 75–88

50. Takeda T, Yu Q, Yuasa T, Hasegawa Y, Yashiro T, Itai Y. Human thyroid specimen imaging by fluorescent x-ray computed tomography with synchrotron radiation. SPIE Proceeding 1999; 3772: 258–267

51. Yu Q, Takeda T, Hasegawa Y, Yuasa T, Itai Y, Akatsuka T. Simultaneous imaging of different contrast materials by fluorescent x-ray computed tomography using synchrotron radiation. Poster abstracts p34–35, 6th International Conference on Biophysics & Synchrotron Radiation (Argonne, USA) August 4–8, 1998

52. Yu Q, Takeda T, Yuasa T, Hasegawa Y, Hyodo K, Dilmanian A, Itai Y, Akatsuka T. Dual elements imaging by fluorescent x-ray computed tomography with synchrotron radiation. J. Synchrotron Rad; submitted

53. Honma S, Sasaki A, Nakai I, Sagai M, Koiso K, Shimojo N. Distribution of copper, selenium, and zinc in human kidney tumors by nondestructive synchrotron radiation x-ray fluorescence imaging. J. of Trace Elements in Experimental Medicine 1993; 6: 163–170

54. Yuasa T, Akiba M, Takeda T, Kazama M, Hoshino Y, Watanabe Y, Hyodo K, Dilmanian FA, Akatsuka T, Itai Y. Reconstruction method for fluorescent x-ray computed tomography by least-squares method using singular value decomposition. IEEE trans. Nucl Sci 1997; 44: 54–62

55. Ando M., Hosoya S. An attempt at X-ray phase-contrast microscopy. Pro. 6th International Conference of X-ray Optics and microanalysis (ed. G. Shinoda, Kohra K, Ichikawa T.) University of Tokyo Press p63–68, 1972

56. Momose A, Fukuda J. Phase-contrast radiographs of nonstained rat cerebellar specimen. Med Phy 1995; 22: 375–379

57. Takeda T, Momose A, Itai Y, Wu J, Hirano K. Phase-contrast imaging with synchrotron x-rays for cancer lesion. Academic Radiology 1995; 2: 799–803

58. Bonse U, Hart M. An X-ray interferometer. Appl Phys Lett 1965; 6: 155–156

59. Forster E, Goetz J, Zaumseil P. Double crystal diffractometry for the characterization of targets for the laser fusion experiments. Krist Tech 1980; 15: 937–945

60. Somenkov VA, Tkalich AK, Shil'shtein S Sh. Refraction contrast in x-ray introscopy. Sov Phys Tech Phys 1991; 36: 1309–1311

61. Davis TJ, Gao D, Gureyev TE, Stevenson AW, Wilkins SW. Phase-contrast imaging of weakly absorbing materials using hard X-rays. Nature 1995a; 373: 595–598

62. Davis TJ, Gureyev TE, Gao D, Stevenson AW, Wilkins SW. X-ray image contrast from a simple phase object. Phys Rev Lett 1995b; 74: 3173–3176

63. Ingal VN, Beliaevskaya EA. X-ray plane-wave topography observation of the phase contrast from a non-crystalline object. J Phys D 1995; 28: 2314–2317

64. Snigirev A. The recent development of Bragg-fresnel crystal optics. Experiments and applications at the ESRF (invited) Rev Sci Instrum 1995; 66: 2053–2058

65. Snigirev A, Snigirev I, Suvorov A, Kocsis M, Kohn V. Phase contrast microimaging by coherent high energy synchrotron radiation. ESRF Newsl 1995b; 24: 23–25

66. Cloetens P, Barratt R, Baruchel J, Guigay JP, Schlenker M. Phase Objects in synchrotron radiation hard x-ray imaging. J Phys D 1996; 29: 133–146

67. Raven C, Snigirev A, Snigireva I, Spanne P, Souvorov A, Kohn V. Phase contrast microtomography with coherent high-energy synchrotron X rays. Appl Phys Lett 1996; 69: 1826–1828

68. Nugent KA, Gureyev TE, Cookson DJ, Paganin D, Barnea Z. Quantitative phase imaging using hard X rays. Phys Rev Lett 1996; 77: 2961–2964

69. Wilkins SW, Gureyev TE, Gao D, Pogany A, Stevenson AW. Phase-contrast imaging using polychromatic hard X rays. Nature 1996; 384: 335–338

70. Snigirev A, Snigirev I, Bosecke P, Lequien S, Schelokov I. High energy X-ray phase contrast microscopy using a circular Bragg-Frenel lens. Opt Commun 1997; 135: 378–384

71. Momose A. Demonstration of phase-contrast X-ray computed tomography using an X-ray interferometer. Nucl Instr Meth 1995; A352: 622–628

72. Momose A, Takeda T, Itai Y, Hirano K. Phase-contrast x-ray computed tomography for observing biological soft tissues. Nature Medicine 1996; 2: 473–475

73. Momose A, Takeda T, Itai Y. Phase-contrast x-ray computed tomography for observing biological specimens and organic materials. Rev Sci Instrum 1995; 66: 1434–1436

74. Momose A, Takeda T, Itai Y, Hirano K. Tomographic image reconstruction using x-ray phase information. SPIE Proceeding 1996; 2708: 674–684

75. Beckmann F, Bonse U, Busck F, Gunnewig O. X-ray microtomography using phase contrast for the investigation of organic matter. J Computer Assisted Tomography 1997; 21: 539–553

76. Momose A, Takeda T, Itai Y, Hirano K. X-ray microscopy and spectromicroscopy. Edited by Thieme J, Schmahl G, Umbach E, Rudolph D, pII/207–212, Springer-Verlag, Heidelberg, 1998

77. Takeda T, Momose A, Ueno E, Itai Y. Phase-contrast x-ray CT image of breast tumor. J Synchrotron Rad. 1998; 5: 1133–1135

78. Momose A, Takeda T, Itai Y. Phase-contrast x-ray computed tomography for biological imaging. SPIE Proceeding 1997; 3149: 120–129

79. Takeda T, Momose A, Hirano K, Haraoka S, Watanabe T, Itai Y. Human carcinoma: Early experience with phase-contrast X-ray CT with synchrotron radiation : Comparative specimen study with optical microscopy. Radiology 2000; 214: 298-301

80. Momose A, Takeda T, Itai Y, Tu J, Hirano K. Recent observations with phase-contrast x-ray computed tomography. SPIE Proceeding 1999; 3772: 188–195

81. Sasaki S. X-ray absorption coefficients of the elements (Li to Bi, U. KEK report 90–16 (National Laboratory for High Energy Physics)), 1990

82. Momose A, Takeda T, Itai Y. Contrast effect of blood on phase-contrast x-ray imaging. Academic Radiology 1995; 2: 883–887

83. Takeda T, Momose A, Yu Q, Wu J, Hirano K, Itai Y.: Phase-contrast x-ray imaging with a large monolithic x-ray interferometer. J Synchrotron Rad. 2000; 7: 280–282

84. Becker P. A two-crystal interferometer from different pieces of silicon material. J Appl Cryst 1974; 7: 593–598

85. Momose A, Yoneyama A, Takeda T, Itai Y, Tu J, Hirano K. Project for application of phase-contrast X-ray imaging to medicine using an X-ray interferometer. SPIE Proceedings. 1999; 3770: 23-31

86. Momose A, Yoneyama A, Hirano K. Operation of a two-crystal x-ray interferometer at the Photon Factory. J Synchrotron Rad 1997; 4: 311–312

87. Momose A, Takeda T, Itai Y, Yoneyama A, Hirano K. Phase-contrast tomographic imaging using an x-ray interferometer. J Synchrotron Rad 1998; 5: 309–314

88. Momose A, Hirano K. The possibility of phase-contrast x-ray microtomography. Jpn J appl Phys 1999; 38: 625-629

7

The molecular basis of inherited skin disorders

M. Giles S. Dunnill   Irene M. Leigh

Considerable advances have been made in the understanding of inherited skin diseases as a result of the wider availability of new molecular laboratory techniques. Genetic disorders in which the gene defect results in a defective structural protein within the epidermis or dermal–epidermal junction form a large part of this chapter. Progress in this area has greatly strengthened the understanding of the molecular anatomy of the skin. The discovery of gene defects in more complex functional genes (some of which were hitherto unknown to have an important role in skin) is now contributing to the field of epithelial cell biology.

Inherited skin disorders are normally classified into one of four types (Table 7.1). Each of these types will be discussed in this chapter.

Table 7.1 Classification of inherited skin disorders

1. Disorders of keratinization	Epidermal keratins
	Loricrin
	Transglutaminase 1
	Fatty aldehyde dehydrogenase
	Steroid sulphatase
2. Desmosomal disorders	Plakophilin 1
	Desmoplakin
	Desmoglein 1
	Sarco/endoplasmic reticulum Ca^{2+} – ATPase type 2 (SERCA2)
3. Gap junction disorders	Connexin 31
	Connexin 26
4. Basement membrane disorders	Plectin
	Type XVII collagen
	Alpha 6 beta 4 integrins
	Laminin 5
	Type VII collagen

M. Giles S. Dunnill MD, MRCP, Consultant Dermatologist, Bristol Royal Infirmary, Marlborough St, Bristol, BS2 8HW, UK

Irene M. Leigh MD FRCP, Professor of Dermatology, Centre for Cutaneous Research, St Bartholomews and the Royal London School of Medicine and Dentistry, Queen Mary and Westfield College, Clinical Sciences and Research Centre, 2 Newark St, London E1 2AT, UK.

KERATIN GENES AND KERATINIZATION

The cutaneous epidermis is comprised principally of keratinocytes (Fig. 7.1). These cells contain intermediate filaments, thought to provide structural strength within the cytoplasm, and confer a degree of flexibility. Intermediate filaments are visible ultrastructurally and can be seen to interact with the cell membrane via hemidesmosomes and desmosomes (Fig. 7.2). At a molecular level, these filaments are composed of keratins.

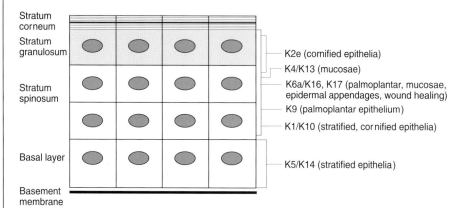

Fig. 7.1 Schematic diagram of keratin expression in epithelium. The expression pattern of different keratins is shown. K5/K14 and K1/K10 are expressed in all squamous epithelia. K9 is confined to palmoplantar epithelium. K6a / K16 are constitutively expressed in palmoplantar epithelium, mucosae, nail bed and hair follicles. They are also expressed during the wound healing response. K17 is limited to palmoplantar and appendageal epithelia. K4/K13 are expressed in mucosae only. K2e is expressed in cornified epithelia. Only those discussed in this chapter are shown.

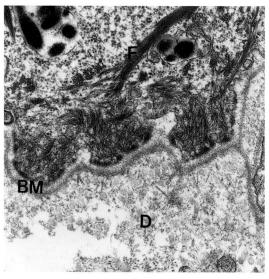

Fig. 7.2 Electron micrograph of dermal–epidermal junction (courtesy of Dr J. A. McGrath). Keratin filaments within the basal cell are visible as bundles of tonofilaments, and appear to interact with the basal plasma membrane in the region of the hemidesmosomes, visible as electron dense plaques on the cytoplasmic surface of the plasma membrane. F, keratin filaments; BM, epidermal basement membrane; D, dermis. (Magnification × 30 000)

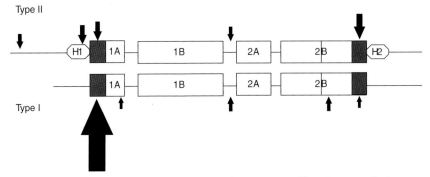

Fig. 7.3 Schematic diagram of the basic molecular structure of keratin. H1 and H2 are variable head and tail domains. There are 4 rod domains: 1A, 1B, 2A and 2B, represented by the boxes. There are highly conserved sequences within the 1A and 2B domains, thought to be important for molecular interactions. The arrows show the sites of mutations in various keratin gene diseases. The size of the arrows indicates the number of mutations reported.

The keratins are a family of intermediate filament proteins of which there are more than 30 subtypes.[1] They are expressed within the cytoplasm of epithelial cells. They all share the same basic molecular structure with a central α-helical rod domain, and non-helical head and tail domains (Fig. 7.3). They are usually expressed in pairs: type I or acidic keratins, and type II or basic keratins. Keratin pairs associate as heterodimers with the central rod domains forming a coiled coil structure. These dimers in turn aggregate in large numbers to form filaments. The highly conserved regions of the helix initiation and helix termination peptides are thought to be important for heterodimer formation and for interaction of keratin filament polymers. Different subtypes of keratin pairs are expressed in a tissue-specific fashion, some being specific for hair follicles, nails or mucous membranes or particular regions of the body such as palmoplantar skin. They may also be expressed within specific layers of the epidermis or in response to wound healing (Fig. 7.1).

Keratinization is a term used to denote terminal differentiation of keratinocytes and the formation of the stratum corneum. This process relates to a number of epithelial cytoskeletal and envelope proteins, glycoproteins and intercellular lipids, but as the name suggests, keratin is the principal molecule involved.

Clinically, inherited disorders of keratin or keratinization include the ichthyoses where the skin is dry, scaly, thickened or flakey. Hair, nails and mucous membranes may be affected. Skin blistering may be a feature. Some of the group of disorders termed ectodermal dysplasias also have clinical features that have classed them as disorders of keratinization.

The following section will start with a discussion of inherited keratin gene diseases, followed by other genes involved in keratinization.

EVIDENCE FOR THE STRUCTURAL ROLE OF KERATINS: MUTATIONS IN KERATIN GENES

Although much evidence has accumulated regarding the structural cytoskeletal function of keratins, the first direct evidence was provided by the discovery that mutations of the basal cell-specific keratin genes resulted in cytolysis of the epidermal basal layer and skin blistering. These mutations were described in patients suffering from Dowling–Meara epidermolysis bullosa simplex.[2,3] This autosomal dominant disease is characterized by blistering of the skin and mucous membranes in response to minor mechanical trauma. Affected children present at or soon after birth with blisters or erosions, and the condition can be life-threatening in the neonatal period due to sepsis. Ultrastructurally keratin filaments of the basal epidermal keratinocytes lack normal filament organization, and appear clumped. Immunoelectron microscopic studies showed that these filament clumps contained the basal cell-specific keratins, 5 and 14.[4] Basal cells may lyse and blister formation occurs through the basal layer. These observations suggested that the primary defect was an abnormality of either keratin 5 (K5) or keratin 14 (K14). At the molecular level, genetic mutations resulting in single amino acid residue substitutions were detected within the highly conserved helix initiation or helix termination peptides of keratins K5 and K14.[2,3] Thus the prediction that the conserved amino acid residue sequences within the helix boundary peptides were vital for filament assembly was supported by clinical and ultrastructural observations in patients with disruptive mutations. This pattern of mutation has now been demonstrated in many different keratin genes with similar cytoskeletal consequences.

THE TISSUE-SPECIFIC DISTRIBUTION OF KERATINS IS MIRRORED BY THE PHENOTYPE

EPIDERMOLYSIS BULLOSA SIMPLEX VARIANTS: DIFFERENT TYPES OF KERATIN K5 / K14 MUTATION

Whilst Dowling–Meara epidermolysis bullosa simplex (EBS) has a severe phenotype, there are two other EBS variants with less severe clinical features. Autosomal dominant Webber–Cockayne EBS is a variant in which children may not manifest the disease until they are fully mobile, and blistering is largely confined to sites of maximum friction such as the palms and soles. Basal cell cytolysis results in blisters, but keratin filament clumps are not seen ultrastructurally. The disease is caused by missense mutations in keratins K5 and K14, but not within the helix boundary peptides. Mutations so far described have been within the L12 linker region and less highly conserved regions of the rod domain.[5] The functional implication is that these regions are less important for filament assembly, but nonetheless have some role.

EBS–Koebner is a rare autosomal recessive condition in which generalized epidermal blisters occur spontaneously or after minor friction. Ultrastructurally, intact basal keratinocytes are remarkable for a complete absence of keratin filaments. Homozygous premature termination codon mutations in keratin K14 have been shown to underlie this variant.[6] The result is a complete absence of K14 on immunostaining, and although K5 is present, it is unable to form filamentous structures. This keratin gene 'knockout' mutation is remarkable in that all other keratin gene mutations described are amino acid residue substitution missense mutations. Interestingly K14 gene knockout mutations in mice have been investigated using gene targeting, but the clinical consequences are not identical, perhaps due to different mechanisms of compensation for the absent protein.[7]

PALM AND SOLE SPECIFIC KERATIN GENE MUTATIONS UNDERLIE THE PALMOPLANTAR KERATODERMAS

In palmoplantar keratoderma (PPK), a biopsy of involved skin may or may not show evidence of cell lysis and tissue separation, allowing subtyping of PPK into epidermolytic and non-epidermolytic. Epidermolytic PPK can occur as part of the syndrome of epidermolytic hyperkeratosis, but also occurs alone as a distinct autosomal dominant clinical entity, sometimes referred to as Vorner's palmoplantar keratoderma. Ultrastructural examination of palm or sole skin reveals suprabasal keratin filament clumping and cell lysis, and the underlying mutations occur in the conserved helix boundary peptides of keratin K9.[8]

A number of other hereditary palmoplantar keratodermas without epidermolysis have been described. Focal non-epidermolytic palmoplantar keratoderma has been shown to result from missense mutations within the helix initiation peptides of keratin K16.[9] Ultrastructurally there is no keratin filament clumping or epidermolysis, but clinical examination of affected family members can reveal orogenital hyperkeratosis and very subtle nail changes, correlating with the known tissue distribution of this keratin. The epidermal expression patterns of keratins 9 and 16 are similar within palm and sole skin, so the differences in phenotype produced by similar distruptive mutations of these two keratins presumably reflects subtle differences in function.

EPIDERMOLYTIC HYPERKERATOSIS AND ICHTHYOSIS BULLOSA OF SIEMENS: MUTATIONS IN THE SUPRABASAL KERATINS K1/K10 AND K2E

Epidermolytic hyperkeratosis (bullous ichthyosiform erythroderma) is an autosomal dominant disease that presents at or soon after birth with erythroderma, widespread skin blistering and erosions. During childhood the phenotype evolves, with a diminished tendency to blistering and the formation of an ichthyotic rippled hyperkeratosis of the skin. Palmoplantar keratoderma (thickening of the palms and soles) is a prominant feature. Ultrastructurally, keratin filaments are clumped and cell lysis is visible in suprabasal keratinocytes. Deleterious amino acid residue substitutions have been reported within the conserved helix boundary peptides of the differentiation-specific keratins, K1 and K10.[10] The suprabasal pattern of expression of these keratins corresponds to the site of primary epidermal pathology.

Ichthyosis bullosa of Siemens is a disease that was originally thought to be a milder variant of epidermolytic hyperkeratosis. There is no erythroderma, and although blistering can occur in response to trauma, it is superficial and more often erosions or 'moulting' of the skin result. The distribution of skin lesions is predominantly flexural, and other areas of the skin may be normal. Electron microscopy of the epidermis reveals keratin filament clumping, but this is confined to the granular and upper spinous layers of the epidermis, where cytolysis can also occur. Thus there are clear clinical and pathological distinctions between this disease and bullous ichthyosiform erythroderma. Keratin gene mutations underlying this disease were defined within the conserved helix boundary peptides of the differentiation specific epidermal keratin K2e, which is expressed only in the upper layers of the epidermis.[11] Thus the subtle differences between these two diseases can be explained precisely by an understanding of the different epidermal expression patterns of the two keratin genes involved.

MUTATIONS IN KERATINS K6A, K16 AND K17: PACHYONYCHIA CONGENITA

Pachyonychia congenita is an autosomal dominant ectodermal dysplasia that is conventionally divided into two subtypes on the basis of clinical features. All patients suffer from characteristic hypertrophic nail dystrophy and nail bed hyperkeratosis. The Jadassohn–Lewandowsky variant (PC-I) is characterized in addition by focal palmoplantar hyperkeratosis, follicular keratoses and oral leukokeratoses. Whereas the Jackson–Lawlor phenotype (PC-II) lacks oral lesions, but includes multiple epidermal follicular cysts (steatocysts), hair abnormalities and natal teeth. Mutations within the conserved helix initiation peptides of keratins K6a and K16 have been shown to underlie PC-I and those of K17 to underlie PC-II.[12,13] The different expression patterns of K6a/K16 compared with K17 elegantly correlate with the clinical phenotypes of their respective pacyonychia congenita variants (see Fig. 7.1).

Keratin 17 mutations have also been identified in two families suffering from steatocystoma multiplex, an autosomal dominant condition featuring multiple cutaneous cysts. The authors of this report evaluated the nails of affected patients, and a number of them had subtle changes.[14] Thus steatocystoma multiplex may be a variant of PC-II. Similarly, non-epidermolytic PPK may be viewed as a *forme fruste* of PC-I. To date all mutations described in patients within this group of disorders have occurred in the helix boundary peptides of keratins K6a, K16 and K17, but presumably the amino acid residue substitutions in patients with PC-I or PC-II are more disruptive to keratin filament formation than in focal non-epidermolytic palmoplantar keratoderma and steatocystoma multiplex respectively, leading to a more extensive phenotype.

KERATINS K4 AND K13 ARE MUCOUS-MEMBRANE SPECIFIC: MUTATIONS CAUSE WHITE SPONGE NAEVUS

Mucosal hyperkeratotic plaques with a spongy appearance give this autosomal dominant condition its name. Plaques occur most commonly in the mouth, but also in the nose, oesophagus and ano-genital mucosa. Electron microscopy of areas of hyperkeratosis again reveal keratin filament aggregation within the cytoplasm of keratinocytes of the spinous layers reflecting similar pathology to other keratin gene disorders. Mutations have recently been described within the helix initiation peptide of keratins K3 and K14, which are expressed in suprabasal mucosal epithelia.[15,16]

MUTATIONS IN GENES OF EPIDERMAL DIFFERENTIATION UNDERLIE ICHTHYOSES AND ECTODERMAL DYSPLASIAS

Besides keratin, terminal differentiation of stratified squamous epithelia involves a number of other molecules. As keratinocytes differentiate in the upper granular layer, they become anucleate cornified cells forming laminated sheets in the stratum corneum. Cytoplasmic keratin filaments are aligned into macrofibres stabilized by disulphide bonds under the influence of fillaggrin, a protein synthesized in the granular layer. Involucrin, loricrin and small proline-rich proteins are related proteins that form a highly insoluble cornified cell envelope within the plasma membrane of the corneocyte. Epidermal transglutaminase catalyses lysine cross-linking of these proteins. Lipids derived from lamellar granules also play an important part in the skin barrier. Desquamation of the outer layer of the stratum corneum requires breakdown of intercellular lipids under the action of steroid sulphatase. Specific mutations have now been identified in a number of the genes governing terminal differentiation, resulting in various ichthyotic phenotypes.

MUTATIONS OF LORICRIN RESULT IN VOHWINKEL'S KERATODERMA

Patients with this autosomal dominant condition suffer from a 'honeycomb' hyperkeratosis of the palms and soles. In addition they may develop characteristic constricting bands around the digits of the hands and feet, known as pseudoainhum, which can lead to autoamputation, especially of the fifth digit. Starfish-shaped hyperkeratotic lesions may also occur on the knuckles and dorsum of the hands. The histological findings are a markedly thickened stratum corneum, hypergranulosis and hyperkeratosis with the hallmark feature of round nuclei retained in the stratum corneum. This disease was shown to be caused by defects within the loricrin gene when a heterozygous frameshift mutation was found in one family affected with this disease.[17] This mutation resulted in a delayed termination codon and mistranslation of the terminal 84 amino acid residues. The region of the protein disrupted by this mutation is thought to be involved in lysine cross-linkage by transglutaminase. Thus the abnormal loricrin protein in these patients' skin is thought to incorporate less efficiently into the cornified cell envelope and to accumulate in intranuclear granules.

TRANSGLUTAMINASE-1 GENE MUTATIONS CAUSE LAMELLAR ICHTHYOSIS

Autosomal recessive lamellar ichthyosis is a severe skin disorder often presenting at birth with a 'collodion' membrane. After this membrane is shed, infants suffer life-long generalized severe ichthyosis with large scales and variable erythroderma. The molecular defects underlying a subgroup of these diseases are disruptive mutations of the keratinocyte transglutaminase gene (TGK, transglutaminase 1). These mutations cause reduced espression of TGK and loss of TGK activity.[18] The resulting clinical phenotype with epidermal thickening and scales attests to the importance of this enzyme in the formation of cornified cell envelope and keratinization. Recent genetic linkage studies have demonstrated a second locus for lamellar ichthyosis on chromosome 2q33-35, and have also shown that some families are non-linked to either this locus or the TGK-1 locus on chromosome 14q.[19] Thus there are at least three loci for this disorder.

MUTATIONS AFFECTING LIPID METABOLISM CAN CAUSE SOME FORMS OF ICHTHYOSIS

X-linked ichthyosis is one of the most common X-linked disorders, and is due to an inborn error of metabolism resulting in steroid sulphatase deficiency. Patients may be born post-term due to low placental oestriol production. Ichthyosis usually starts in the first year with dry brown scaly skin. The underlying molecular defect in many patients has been shown to be a total gene deletion of the steroid sulphatase gene on the X chromosome.[20] Over 80% of patients harbour steroid sulphatase gene deletions. Because of the proximity of the steroid sulphatase gene to the genes for Kallman syndrome and short stature, patients may suffer from these diseases as well, as a result of a contiguous gene defect.[21] In those patients where no gene deletion can be detected, the steroid sulphatase protein is still absent, but the exact nature of the genetic defect is unclear. It may involve deleterious point mutations of the steroid sulphatase gene, or mutations affecting post-translational modification.

Sjogren–Larsson syndrome is an autosomal recessive condition characterized by mental retardation, spasticity and severe generalized ichthyosis. The ichthyosis presents at or soon after birth, but the neurological symptoms are not evident until the first or second year of life. Patients are deficient in fatty aldehyde dehydrogenase, an enzyme which catalyses the oxidation of long-chain aliphatic aldehydes to fatty acids.[22] This is part of the metabolic pathway for oxidation of fatty alcohols, and affected patients have raised fatty alcohol levels in plasma. Deleterious mutations have now been described in the fatty aldehyde dehydrogenase gene encoding this enzyme. The mechanism of ichthyosis is unclear, but probably relates to deranged lipid metabolism in the stratum corneum and central nervous system, with accumulation of fatty alcohol.

DESMOSOMAL DISORDERS

Desmosomes are visible ultrastructurally as electon-dense arrangements at the cell membrane where two adjacent cells join. Inner and outer plaques are discernible on both sides of the junction. Desmosomes act as an anchoring point for the keratin filaments to the cell membrane, and for one cell cytoskeleton to the next. Structural proteins that make up desmosomes interact directly or indirectly with keratin filaments at the molecular level. These proteins include desmosomal cadherins (desmogleins and desmocollins), desmosomal plaque proteins (desmoplakin and plakoglobin) and the accessory plaque protein, plakophilin 1. Direct evidence for the role of these proteins in molecular conjunction at the cell–cell interface has come from the inherited dermatoses described below.

MUTATIONS IN THE DESMOSOMAL PROTEIN, PLAKOPHILIN 1, INDUCE AN ECTODERMAL DYSPLASIA WITH SKIN FRAGILITY

This autosomal recessive disorder has recently been described, and has features of a skin blistering disorder with abnormalities of hair, nails and sweat glands. Hyperkeratosis, scaling and cracking of the skin develops, especially on the palms and soles. Microscopic examination of skin reveals loss of cell–cell adhesion within the epidermis (acantholysis), thus the skin blistering does not arise from cell lysis as occurs in the keratin gene disorders. A compound heterozygous null allele mutation in the gene for plakophilin 1 has been found in affected patients.[23,24] This resulted in an absence of immunodetectable plakophilin 1 in the patients' skin. Plakophilin 1 localizes to the desmosomes at cell–cell junctions throughout the spinous layers of stratified squamous epithelia, and is thought to mediate intermediate filament/desmosome interaction. It may also have a role in signal transduction and thus an effect on cell behaviour during development. The clinical and pathological features of the patient reported provide strong evidence that this protein has a role in cutaneous cell–cell adhesion and imply that it has a role in epidermal morphogenesis.

STRIATE PALMOPLANTAR KERATODERMA MAY BE CAUSED BY MUTATIONS WITHIN THE GENES FOR DESMOPLAKIN OR DESMOGLEIN 1

Striate palmoplantar keratoderma is a clinically distinct subtype of focal keratoderma characterized by linear skin thickening over the flexor aspects of the fingers and palms. Focal areas of thickening are also found on the soles. Inheritance is autosomal dominant. There are no consistent associated features, although one report documents hair, nail and dental abnormalities in addition. Genetic heterogeneity was shown in separate studies that found linkage to 18q21 in one kindred and to 6p21 in another. Investigation of the locus on 18q21 revealed a mutation within the gene encoding the desmosomal cadherin, desmoglein 1.[25] The heterozygous mutation described resulted in deletion of part of the extracellular domain of desmoglein 1, known to be involved in molecular interactions. The mutant protein could act in a dominant negative fashion, incorporating into and disrupting desmosomes. Alternatively the mutant protein could remain in the cytoplasm and sequester other desmosomal proteins such as plakoglobin or plakophilin 1.

The gene for the desmosomal plaque protein, desmoplakin, maps to 6p21 and a mutation resulting in haplo-insufficiency of this protein has recently been described in a kindred with striate palmoplantar keratoderma.[26] Desmoplakin lacks a transmembrane domain and also has a putative role in linking cytoplasmic intermediate filaments to the cell membrane at desmosomes. Ultrastructural examination of desmosomes in an affected individual showed poorly-formed cytoplasmic inner plaques and lack of desmosome–keratin filament interaction.

DARIER DISEASE IS AN ACANTHOLYTIC DISORDER CAUSED BY DISRUPTION OF THE CA^{2+} PUMP GENE, ATP2A2

Darier disease exhibits abnormal keratinization and has features of a desmosomal disorder. It is included here because the characteristic histological finding is acantholysis, although it could equally be discussed in the section on disorders of keratinization.

The clinical features of this autosomal dominant genodermatosis are warty papules and plaques over the seborrhoeic areas of the skin, palmoplantar pits and characteristic nail dystrophy. In some kindreds neuropsychiatric abnormalities such as mental retardation and epilepsy also occur. Ultrastructural studies demonstrate desmosomal abnormalities with loss of keratin–desmosome attachments, suggesting that the underlying defect relates to the adhesion molecules of the desmosomes. A positional cloning approach resulted in the identification of disruptive mutations within the ATP2A2 gene, which encodes the sarco/endoplasmic reticulum Ca^{2+}-ATPase type 2 isoform (SERCA2).[27] This Ca^{2+} pump protein is involved in intracellular Ca^{2+} signalling. The assembly of epithelial cell desmosomes *in vitro* has been shown to be dependent on fluctuations in extracellular Ca^{2+} concentration. Variation of intracellular Ca^{2+} concentration may also be important in regulation of cell–cell adhesion. Thus, although the exact pathogenic mechanism in Darier disease is uncertain, there are clear indications that SERCA2 disruption impairs desmosome assembly or alters anchorage of keratin filaments to desmosomal plaques.

DISORDER OF GAP JUNCTIONS

MUTATIONS OF THE CONNEXIN 31 GENE GJB3 CAUSE ERYTHROKERATODERMA VARIABILIS

The autosomal dominant dermatosis erythrokeratoderma variabilis exhibits variable expression within families and within individuals. Two types of skin lesion occur: fixed, dark, erythematous, hyperkeratotic plaques on extensor surfaces and polycyclic, migratory, erythematous macules. The disease was originally linked to the Rhesus locus on 1p and has now been shown to be caused by mutations within the gene encoding connexin 31, a gap junction protein.[28] Connexins assemble into hexameric transmembrane structures forming pores of communication between adjacent cells. These areas of communication, termed gap junctions, are visible under electron microscopic examination and are believed to play an important role in intercellular signaling. How disruption of connexin 31 function leads to the skin phenotype in erythrokeratoderma variabilis is as yet unclear.

MUTATIONS OF CONNEXIN 26 GJB2 CAUSE VOHWINKEL'S KERATODERMA

Following a study of a family with hereditary sensorineural deafness and Vohwinkel's keratoderma, where multiple mutations in GB2+3 have been reported,[29] there has been widespread acceptance throughout the literature that recessive sensorineural deafness results from mutations in GBJ2 encoding connexin 26. Dominant mutations in GBJ2 (connexin 26) can also cause hereditary sensorineural deafness on a background of other connexin mutations. However, one particular mutation in GBJ2 (D66H) causes Vohwinkel's keratoderma. The location of point mutations in connexin 26, all believed to result in changes in voltage gating, therefore appears critical in the causation of keratoderma and hereditary deafness.

DISORDERS OF THE EPITHELIAL BASEMENT MEMBRANE ZONE

THE EPIDERMAL BASEMENT MEMBRANE ZONE AS A CHAIN OF ADHESION MOLECULES

The basement membrane between the cutaneous epidermis and dermis has several functions. It acts as a barrier and a gateway for molecules passing between the two zones, and also serves to attach the keratinocytes of the epidermis to the connective tissue within the dermis. Disruption of the second of these functions leads to disorders in which blistering and erosions arise in the skin and mucous membranes.

Much of our understanding of the anatomy of the basement membrane zone was initially derived from electron microscopy studies.[30] Hemidesmosomes, electron dense structures along the basement membrane, are thought to act as adhesion zones, linking keratin filaments of the basal keratinocytes to dermal collagen bundles (Fig. 7.2). Many structural proteins have been localized in the vicinity of hemidesmosomes, and may act as links in a dermal–epidermal molecular chain (Fig. 7.4). Direct evidence for the importance of many of these molecules has now been gained from the study of inherited skin blistering diseases in which molecular genetic mutations have been defined. Gene targeting in animal model systems has yielded further important information regarding individual molecules.[31]

EPIDERMOLYSIS BULLOSA IS AN HERIDITARY SKIN BLISTERING DISEASE COMPRISING VARIOUS SUBTYPES

Patients with epidermolysis bullosa (EB) suffer from blistering of the skin after minor mechanical trauma.[32] This can vary in severity such that some groups of patients have a generalized tendency to blister after light friction on the skin, whereas others only blister in localized body sites after more severe rubbing. EB has been divided into three subtypes on the basis of the exact ultrastructural level of dermal–epidermal separation. In dystrophic EB separation occurs below the lamina densa of the epidermal basement membrane; in junctional EB the level is within the lamina lucida; and with EB simplex the separation occurs within the basal keratinocytes of the epidermis (Fig. 7.4).

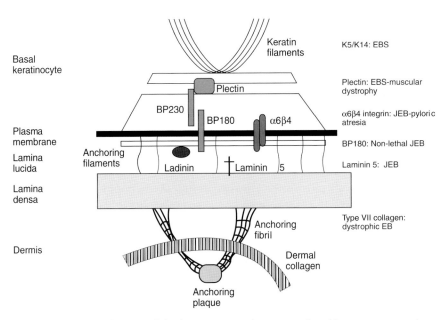

Fig. 7.4 Schematic diagram of the basement membrane zone/hemidesmosome complex. Hemidesmosomes are visible ultrastructurally as electron dense plaques along the basal plasma membrane of the keratinocyte (see Fig. 7.2). The locations of structural proteins within the hemidesmosomes, the lamina lucida, and below the lamina densa are shown. The exact molecular interaction of each of these proteins is still unclear, but there is some evidence that many of these proteins link with each other, or with as yet undescribed molecules, to form a structural chain linking the keratin filaments of the basal keratinocyte to the dermal collagen. EBS, epidermolysis bullosa simplex; JEB, junctional epidermolysis bullosa.

DYSTROPHIC EB MAY BE AUTOSOMAL DOMINANT OR RECESSIVE AND MAY VARY GREATLY IN CLINICAL SEVERITY

Dystrophic EB patients may suffer scarring after blistering and nail, mucous membrane and oesophageal mucosal lesions are common. In general, autosomal recessive inheritance confers a more severe phenotype compared to dominant inheritance. The most severely affected patients are born with erosions over large areas of the body and limbs and may die in infancy. Survival into childhood allows the development of severe scarring deformities such as limb contractures and pseudosyndactyly, and patients suffer chronic non-healing skin erosions. In contrast, affected members of families with mild subtypes may have dystrophic toe nails and minor scarring around the ankles as their only feature. Ultrastructurally skin from affected patients shows varying defects of anchoring fibrils below the lamina densa.[32] These attachment structures are known to be composed of type VII collagen.

BOTH AUTOSOMAL DOMINANT AND RECESSIVE DYSTROPHIC EB ARE CAUSED BY MUTATIONS IN THE TYPE VII COLLAGEN GENE AND PHENOTYPIC VARIATION IS EXPLAINED BY SITE AND TYPE OF MUTATION

Genetic linkage studies using families with autosomal dominant or recessive dystrophic EB prove tight linkage to the type VII collagen gene (COL7A1) at 3p21.[34,35] Patients with dominantly inherited disease harbour glycine substitutions within the collagen helical region of COL7A1.[36] This type of mutation has previously been demonstrated in other collagen gene disorders,[37] and by analogy it is to be expected that exon-skipping mutations within the collagen VII helix will also result in dominant dystrophic EB.

The most severe forms of autosomal recessive dystrophic EB (Hallopeau–Siemens) are caused by COL7A1 mutations resulting in premature termination codons on both alleles.[38] These are shown to exert their effect by instability of messenger RNA and complete absence of type VII collagen protein in skin. The severity of disease caused by the total lack of this molecule attests to the importance of type VII collagen and anchoring fibrils in dermal–epidermal adhesion.

However, not all recessively inherited forms of dystrophic EB are severe. Mutations described in these patients reveal a combination of homozygous missense mutations or compound heterozygous missense/premature termination codon mutations.[39] Genotype–phenotype correlation studies also suggest that the site of the premature termination codon mutation within COL7A1 may also determine disease severity.[40]

JUNCTIONAL EB IS A HETEROGENEOUS DISORDER HIGHLIGHTING ADHESION PROPERTIES OF SEVERAL HEMIDESMOSOMAL MOLECULAR COMPONENTS

Junctional EB patients do not have such a marked tendency to scar compared to dystrophic EB patients, and the phenotype may involve abnormalities of hair and teeth as well as nails. There are two major subtypes, both autosomal recessive. Herlitz or lethal junctional EB is extremely severe with a poor prognosis, the majority of affected patients dying in infancy from sepsis, malnutrition and fluid loss resulting from mucocutaneous erosions. Non-lethal junctional EB is less severe and patients may survive childhood. A particular subtype of non-lethal junctional EB is termed generalized atrophic benign EB and is characterized by sparse hair, atrophic scaring and a better prognosis.

The rarity of these diseases, together with their potential genetic heterogeneity and autosomal recessive inheritance has precluded investigation using genetic linkage. Indirect immunofluorescence studies using antibodies directed against lamina lucida/hemidesmosomal antigens, however, have produced candidate genes for mutational screening. Subgroups of junctional EB patients have been shown to exhibit reduced staining using both laminin 5 (GB3) and bullous pemphigoid antigen 2 antibodies.[41,42] Thus both laminin 5 and bullous pemphigoid antigen 2 were shown to be candidate genes for junctional EB. Laminin 5 is a heterotrimeric non-collagenous protein. The three genes encoding the separate component molecules are LAMA3, LAMB3 and LAMC2, and mutations have been described in all three in junctional EB patients. Homozygous or compound heterozygous premature termination codon mutations occur in LAMA3,[43] LAMB3,[44] and LAMC2.[45] In affected patients, such mutations in one of the laminin 5 genes results in total lack of that particular protein product. The laminin 5 heterotrimer is either unstable or assembly is severely impaired regardless of which gene is mutated.

In less severe non-lethal phenotypes, underlying laminin 5 mutations have been shown to consist of compound heterozygous premature codon (PTC)/missense mutations in a situation analogous to that of COL7A1 in dystrophic EB.[46] In the generalized atrophic benign EB phenotype, compound PTC/missense mutations have been found in LAMB3,[41] but interestingly this phenotype also results from homozygous or compound heterozygous mutations of the bullous pemphigoid antigen 2 gene, BPAG2, also known as COL17A1.[42] Both PTC/PTC and PTC/missense mutations have been described.[47] The conclusions from these observations is that laminin 5 and bullous pemphigoid antigen 2 are closely associated within the lamina lucida.

JUNCTIONAL EB WITH PYLORIC ATRESIA IS CAUSED BY MUTATIONS OF THE α6β4 INTEGRINS COMPLEX

A rare subtype of junctional EB in which infants are born with pyloric atresia has long been recognized. Skin blistering is not always severe, but if patients survive surgical correction of the pyloric obstruction, they may develop uretero-vesical obstruction, possibly as a result of transitional epithelial micro-trauma. Patients with this autosomal recessive disorder have been identified with deleterious compound heterozygous mutations of the β4 integrin gene, ITGB4.[48] Recently, similar mutations have been described in the α6 integrin gene, ITGA6.[49] Integrins are transmembrane proteins that are known to play a role in cell–cell and cell–matrix interactions, and may be involved in the regulation of cell growth. They are expressed as heterodimers, and the α6β4 pair are present within hemidesmosomes of stratified squamous and transitional epithelial basement membranes. Null allele mutations of either ITGA6 or ITGB4 preclude expression of the heterodimer. The EB clinical phenotype suggests that the α6β4 integrin is important for cell–matrix adhesion at the cutaneous basement membrane zone. The mechanism responsible for pyloric atresia in these patients is not yet clear, but repeated prenatal trauma and impaired wound healing at the pylorus has been suggested.[48]

EB SIMPLEX WITH MUSCULAR DYSTROPHY IS CAUSED BY MUTATIONS OF PLECTIN, A CYTOSKELETAL-MEMBRANE ANCHOR PROTEIN

This subtype of EB simplex is unique in that the main clinical feature is a progressive muscular dystrophy and neurological degeneration. Ultrastructural studies of skin suggest that tissue separation occurs within the basal keratinocyte, but the level of separation is just above the basal plasma membrane, making it difficult to distinguish from the lamina lucida split of junctional EB. Indirect immunofluorescence using antibodies to plectin identified this molecule as the candidate protein for this disease. Homozygous and compound heterozygous premature termination codon mutations of the plectin gene have been shown to underlie this disease.[50,51] Plectin is widely distributed in brain, muscle and skin and is thought to anchor cytoskeletal intermediate filaments to the cell membrane. Loss of this function in neuromuscular and cutaneous tissue is reflected in the various clinical features of this disease.

CONCLUSIONS

This chapter has covered the major gene–protein systems relevant to the skin in which the molecular pathology of inherited skin diseases have been described. Many further genetic disorders could have been included by virtue of skin involvement: neurofibromatosis, tuberous sclerosis and oculo-cutaneous albinism to name three. It is also to be expected that the molecular pathology of other inherited skin diseases will be unravelled in the near future. It is fascinating to await these developments and to anticipate the determination of function of previously unrecognized molecular systems within the skin.

KEY POINTS

1. Inherited skin disorders are normally classified into one of four types. The molecular pathology of each type is discussed in this chapter.
2. The first type is the disorders of keratinization, which can be due to mutations in specific keratin genes or to mutations in other genes involved in keratinization.
3. There are more than 30 subtypes of keratin proteins. Many are distributed in specific tissues such as palms, soles, nails etc and the phenotypes of various disorders mirror these tissue-specific distributions.
4. The second type is the desmosomal disorders. These are characterized histologically by a loss of cell–cell adhesion. The different disorders can be characterized phenotypically. Histologically they can be characterized on the basis of the site and type of cell–cell interaction that has been disrupted.
5. Gap junction disorders are the third type and are related to mutations in connexin genes.
6. The fourth category is the basement membrane disorders. The most com-

monly seen phenotypes are inherited skin blistering diseases, in particular the three subtypes of epidermolysis bullosa. Phenotypic variations can be explained by the site and type of genetic mutation.

REFERENCES

1. Lane EB. Keratins. In: Royce PM, Steinmann B (Eds) Connective Tissue and its Heritable Disorders. Molecular, Genetic, and Medical Aspects. New York: Wiley-Liss Inc., 1993; 237–247

2. Coulombe PA, Hutton ME, Letai A et al. Point mutations in human keratin 14 genes of epidermolysis bullosa simplex patients: genetic and functional analysis. Cell 1991; 66: 1301–1311

3. Lane EB, Rugg EL, Navsaria H et al. A mutation in the conserved helix termination peptide of keratin 5 in hereditary skin blistering. Nature 1992; 356: 244–246

4. Ishada-Yamamoto A, McGrath JA, Chapman SJ et al. Epidermolysis bullosa simplex (Dowling–Meara subtype) is a genetic disease characterized by an abnormal keratin filament network involving keratins K5 and K14. J Invest Dermatol 1991; 97: 959–968

5. Rugg EL, Morley SM, Smith FJD et al. Missing links: Weber–Cockayne keratin mutations implicate the L12 linker domain in effective cytoskeleton function. Nature Genet 1993; 5: 294–300

6. Rugg EL, McLean WHI, Lane EB et al. A functional 'knockout' of human keratin 14. Genes Develop 1994; 8: 2563–2573

7. Lloyd C, Yu QC, Cheng J et al. The basal keratin network of stratified squamous epithelia: defining K15 function in the absence of K14. J Cell Biol 1995; 129: 1329–1344

8. Reis A, Hennies H-C, Langbein L et al. Keratin 9 gene mutations in epidermolytic palmoplantar keratoderma (EPPK). Nature Genet 1994; 6: 174–179

9. Shamser MK, Navsaria HA, Stevens HP et al. Novel mutations in keratin 16 gene underly focal non-epidermolytic palmoplantar keratoderma (NEPPK) in two families. Hum Mol Genet 1995; 4: 1875–1881

10. Rothnagel JA, Dominey AM, Dempsey LD et al. Mutations in the rod domains of keratins 1 and 10 in epidermolytic hyperkeratosis. Science 1992; 257: 1128–1130

11. McLean WHI, Morley SM, Lane SM et al. Ichthyosis bullosa of Siemens – a disease involving keratin 2e. J Invest Dermatol 1994; 103: 277–281

12. McLean WHI, Rugg EL, Lunny DP et al. Keratin 16 and keratin 17 mutations cause pachyonychia congenita. Nature Genet 1995; 9: 273–278

13. Bowden PE, Haley JL, Kansky A et al. Mutation of a type II keratin gene (K6a) in pachyonychia congenita. Nature Genet 1995; 10: 363–365

14. Smith FJD, Corden LD, Rugg EL et al. Missense mutations in keratin 17 cause either pachyonychia congenita type 2 or a phenotype resembling steatocystoma multiplex. J Invest Dermatol 1997; 108: 220–223

15. Rugg EL, McLean WHI, Allison WE et al. A mutation in the mucosal keratin K4 is associated with oral white sponge nevus. Nature Genet 1995; 11: 450–452

16. Richard G, De Laurenzi V, Didona B, Bale SJ, Compton JG. Keratin 13 point mutation underlies the hereditary mucosal epithelia disorder white sponge nevus. Nature Genet 1995; 11: 453–455

17. Maestrini E, Monaco AP, McGrath JA et al. A molecular defect in loricrin, the major component of the cornified cell envelope, underlies Vohwinkel's syndrome. Nature Genet 1996; 13: 70–77

18. Huber M, Rettler I, Bernasconi K et al. Mutations of transglutaminase in lamellar ichthyosis. Science 1995; 267: 525–528

19. Parmentier L, Lakhdar H, Blanchet-Bardon C et al. Mapping of a second locus for lamellar ichthyosis to chromosome 2q33–35. Hum Mol Genet 1996; 5: 555–559

20. Ballabio A, Parenti G, Carrozzo R et al. Isolation and characterisation of a steroid sulphatase cDNA clone: genomic deletion in patients with X-linked ichthyosis. Proc Natl Acad Sci USA 1987; 84: 4519–4523

21. Ballabio A, Carrozzo R, Parenti G et al. Molecular heterogeneity of steroid sulphatase deficiency: a multicenter study on 57 unrelated patients, at DNA and protein levels. Genomics 1989; 4: 36–40

22. De Laurenzi V, Rogers GR, Hamrock DJ et al. Sjogren–Larsson syndrome is cause by mutations in the fatty aldehyde dehydrogenase gene. Nature Genet 1996; 12: 52–57

23. McGrath JA, McMillan JA, Shemanko CS et al. Mutations in the plakophilin 1 gene result in ectodermal dysplasia / skin fragility syndrome. Nature Genet 1997; 17: 240–244

24. McGrath JA, Hoeger PH, Christiano AM et al. Skin fragility and hypohidrotic ectodermal dysplasia resulting from ablation of plakophilin 1. Br J Dermatol 1999; 140: 297–307

25. Rickman L, Imrak D, Stevens H et al. Amino-terminal deletion in a desmosomal cadherin causes the skin disease striate palmoplantar keratoderma. Hum Mol Genet 1999; 8: 971–976

26. Keith D, Armstrong B, McKenna KE et al. Haploinsufficiency of desmoplakin causes a striate subtype of plammoplantar keratoderma. Hum Mol Genet 1999; 8: 143–148

27. Sakuntabhai A, Ruiz-Perez V, Carter S et al. Mutations in ATP2A2, encoding a Ca^{2+} pump, cause Darier disease. Nature Genet 1999; 21: 271–277

28. Richard G, Smith LE, Bailey RA et al. Mutations in the human connexin gene GJB3 cause erythrokeratodermia variabilis. Nature Genet 1998; 20: 366–373

29. Kelsell DP, Dunlop J, Stevens HP et al. Connexin 26 mutations in hereditary non-syndromic sensorineural deafness. Nature 1997; 387: 80–82

30. Tidman M J, Eady RAJ. Ultrastructural morphometry of the normal human dermal epidermal junction: the influence of age sex and body region on laminar and non-laminar components. J Invest Dermatol 1984; 83: 448–453

31. Guo L, Degenstein L, Dowling J et al. Gene targeting of BPAG1: abnormalities in mechanical strength and cell migration in stratified epithelia and neurologic degeneration. Cell 1995; 81: 233–243

32. Eady RAJ. Current perspectives and differential diagnosis in epidermolysis bullosa. In: Lin A, Carter M (Eds) Epidermolysis Bullosa. Basic and Clinical Aspects. New York: Springer, 1992; 3–15

33. Tidman MJ, Eady RAJ. Evaluation of anchoring fibrils and other components of the dermo epidermal junction in dystrophic epidermolysis bullosa by a quantitative ultrastructural technique. J Invest Dermatol 1985; 85: 374–377

34. Ryynanen J, Knowlton RJ, Parente MG et al. Human type VII collagen: genetic linkage of the gene (COL7A1) on chromosome 3 to dominant dystrophic epidermolysis bullosa. Am J Hum Genet 1991; 49: 797–803

35. Hovnanian A, Duquesnoy P, Blanchet-Bardon C et al. Genetic linkage of recessive dystrophic epidermolysis bullosa to the type VII collagen gene. J Clin Invest 1992; 90: 1032–1036

36. Christiano AM, Ryynanen M, Uitto J. Dominant dystrophic epidermolysis bullosa: identification of a Gly-Ser substitution in the triple-helical domain of type VII collagen. Proc Natl Acad Sci USA 1994; 91: 3549–3553

37. Prockop DJ. Mutations in collagen genes as a cause of connective tissue disease. New Engl J Med 1992; 326: 540–546

38. Hilal L, Rochat A, Duquesnoy P et al. A homozygous insertion-deletion in the type VII collagen gene (COL7A1) in Hallopeau–Siemens dystrophic epidermolysis bullosa. Nature Genet 1993; 5: 287–293

39. Christiano AM, Greenspan DS, Hoffman GG et al. A missense mutation in type VII collagen in two affected siblings with recessive dystrophic epidermolysis bullosa. Nature Genet. 1993: 4: 62–66

40. Dunnill MGS, McGrath JA, Richards AJ et al. Clinicopathological correlations of compound heterozygous COL7A1 mutations in recessive dystrophic epidermolysis bullosa. J Invest Dermatol 1996; 107: 171–177.

41. McGrath JA, Pulkkinen L, Christiano AM et al. Altered laminin 5 expression due to mutations in the gene encoding the β3 chain (LAMB3) in generalized atrophic benign epidermolysis bullosa. J Invest Dermatol 1995; 104: 467–474

42. McGrath JA, Gatalica B, Christiano AM et al. Mutations in the 180-kD bullous pemphigoid antigen (BPAG2), a hemidesmosomal transmembrane collagen (COL17A1), in generalized atrophic benign epidermolysis bullosa. Nature Genet 1995; 11: 83–86

43. Kivirikko S, McGrath JA, Baudoin C et al. A homozygous nonsense mutation in the α3 chain gene of laminin 5 (LAMA3) in lethal (Herlitz) junctional epidermolysis bullosa. Hum Mol Genet 1995; 4: 959–962

44. Pulkkinen L, Christiano AM, Gerecke DR et al. A homozygous nonsense mutation in the β3 chain gene of laminin 5 (LAMB3) in Herlitz junctional epidermolysis bullosa. Genomics 1994; 24: 357–360

45. Pulkkinen L, Christiano AM, Airenne T et al. Mutations in the γ2 chain gene (LAMC2) of kalinin/laminin 5 in the junctional forms of epidermolysis bullosa. Nature Genet 1994; 6: 293–298

46. McGrath JA, Christiano AM, Pulkkinen L, Eady RAJ, Uitto J. Compound heterozygosity for nonsense and missense mutations in the LAMB3 gene in non-lethal junctional epidermolysis bullosa. J Invest Dermatol 1996; 106: 775–777

47. Darling TN, McGrath JA, Yee C et al. Premature termination codons are present on both alleles of the bullous pemphigoid antigen 2/type XVII collagen gene in five Austrian families with generalized atrophic benign epidermolysis bullosa. J Invest Dermatol 1997; 108: 463–468

48. Vidal F, Aberdam D, Miquel C et al. Integrin β4 mutations associated with junctional epidermolysis bullosa with pyloric atresia. Nature Genet 1995; 10: 229–234

49. Pulkkinen l, Kimonis VE, Xu Y et al. Homozygous alpha6 integrin mutation in junctional epidermolysis bullosa with congenital duodenal atresia. Hum Mol Genet 1997; 6: 669–674

50. Smith FJD, Eady RAJ, Leigh IM et al. Plectin deficiency results in muscular dystrophy with epidermolysis bullosa. Nature Genet 1996; 13: 450–456

51. McLean WHI, Pulkkinen L, Smith FJ et al. Loss of plectin causes epidermolysis bullosa with muscular dystrophy: cDNA cloning and genomic organization. Genes Develop 1996; 10: 1724–1735

8

Routine reporting of non-neoplastic gastric biopsies

Judy Wyatt

INTRODUCTION

The aim of this chapter is to give an overview of the system for categorizing and reporting non-neoplastic biopsies in routine practice. An algorithm for this is given in Fig. 8.1. Some degree of aetiological or clinicopathological diagnosis beyond non-specific chronic gastritis can be given in the large majority of gastric biopsies.

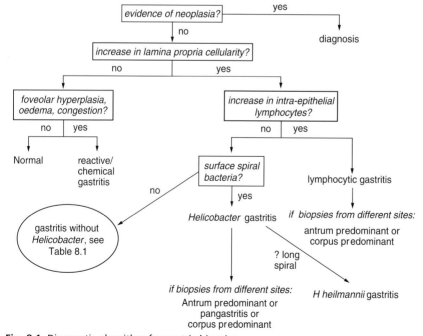

Fig. 8.1 Diagnostic algorithm for gastric biopsies.

Judy Wyatt MBChB FRCPath, Consultant Pathologist, St James's University Hospital, Beckett Street, Leeds LS9 7TF, UK

In this chapter I have included those aspects of gastritis that are of relevance and interest to the histopathologist, to make the task of tackling a pile of gastric biopsies more enjoyable. Diagnosis of gastric neoplasia has not been addressed in this chapter, but is the most important function of gastric biopsy diagnosis.

The recognition of the role of *Helicobacter pylori* in gastric pathology expanded the focus of gastroenterologists and histopathologists beyond the diagnosis of neoplasia in the stomach. Until the 1980s, the goal of endoscopists was to use the improving technology of their endoscopes to find focal lesions (ulcers, cancer) and then to use histology to distinguish them. The exceptions were isolated groups, most notably in Finland and South America, who had studied the progressions of inflammation and atrophy over decades.

Helicobacter pylori was first cultured in 1982,[1] and its high prevalence and involvement in nearly all gastric pathology gradually became recognized over the following decade. Peptic ulcers and gastric cancer develop against a background of a diffuse mucosal field change, and interest in gastric histopathology expanded to include characterization of the gastric mucosa away from the focal lesion. To some, endoscopy was incomplete without biopsy for the histological diagnosis of gastritis. Consequently studies of systematically obtained biopsies allowed the topography and morphology of gastritis to be set in a clinicopathological context, and a new system for classifying these changes (Sydney System[2] and subsequent modification[3]) emerged as a terminology for describing groups of features in the histopathology report.

NORMAL GASTRIC MUCOSA

Anatomical regions of antrum, corpus and cardia are recognizable by their histology.[4] 'Junctional' type mucosa occurs at their boundaries, with parietal cells being frequent among otherwise typical antral glands. The normal gastric lamina propria, unlike other sites in the gastrointestinal tract, contains virtually no plasma cells; occasional aggregates of lymphocytes may be present. The exception is the cardia mucosa, at the gastro-oesophageal junction in which some lamina propria mononuclear cells are normally present. Absence of a physiological mucosa-associated lymphoid tissue was not appreciated in older text books where 'normal gastric mucosa' would now be considered to be an example of gastritis.[5] The concept of this mucosa-associated lymphoid tissue (MALT) acquired in response to stimulation by bacterial antigens, is important in understanding the pathogenesis of gastric lymphoma.

HELICOBACTER GASTRITIS

Members of the genus *Helicobacter* establish long-term stable colonization of gastric (and sometimes other) mucosal surfaces in a variety of animal species.[6] The specificity of each *Helicobacter* species for its particular animal host suggests co-evolution. World-wide the majority of human stomachs harbour *Helicobacter pylori*. Infection usually occurs unrecognized in childhood, persists for decades, and only a minority of infected people will ever present with complications of ulcer or malignancy.

Acute *Helicobacter* gastritis has been recognized only rarely.[7] The initial phase of cytopathic epithelial changes and neutrophil infiltration (when *H. pylori* may not be visible histologically) progresses to the familiar chronic gastritis within a couple of weeks. Subsequently, *Helicobacter* gastritis varies among individuals in its topography and severity, in a way that probably depends on the interplay of four factors: bacterial strain, genetic background of host, other environmental factors and age at which infection occurred. For the histopathologist, biopsies from antrum and corpus mucosa allow the patient to be placed within an overall spectrum of *Helicobacter* gastritis, which has relevance to the risk of complications of the infection (Fig. 8.2).

Chronic gastritis is recognized by an increase in mononuclear cells, particularly plasma cells in the lamina propria. *Helicobacter* infection (current or previous) is by far the commonest cause. *Helicobacter* can be seen on routine haematoxylin and eosin (H & E) stain when numerous, but are more reliably recognized with other histochemical stains, which accentuate their distinctive uniform, curved or wavy morphology, and association with the epithelial cell surface (Fig. 8.3). The use of a stain in addition to H & E improves the accuracy of detection, especially where bacterial load is low, or where other bacteria are present in patients with hypochlorhydria. Giemsa[8] is the most commonly used stain, being simple to perform and reliable, but alternatives exist. Silver stains (Warthin Starry, Genta[9]) give clear results, but are too technically demanding for routine use.

The degree of chronic inflammatory cell infiltration is very variable, as is the degree to which associated features of neutrophil infiltration of the epithelium (activity), glandular atrophy and intestinal metaplasia are present. All of these features can be graded (e.g. from 0–3 in the Sydney System [2,3]); this is useful in research but grading is not necessary for clinical management of the individual patient. Following successful treatment of *Helicobacter,* the activity of gastritis disappears within a few days. Chronic inflammatory infiltrate gradually reduces

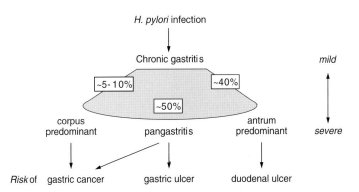

Fig. 8.2 Spectrum of *H. pylori* gastritis. The severity of chronic inflammation and degree of atrophy in different regions of the stomach determine the topographical pattern of gastritis. The more severe gastritis is seen in patients infected with cytotoxin producing strains (Cag A positive strains) of *H. pylori*, and may also depend on environmental factors. The distribution of gastritis is probably determined more by the host's genetic background, and perhaps age of acquisition of *H. pylori*. Percentages of antrum predominant, pangastritis and corpus predominant gastritis are approximate and will vary with the population studied.

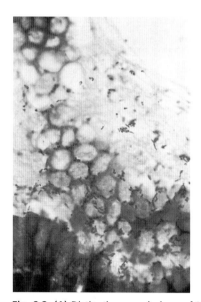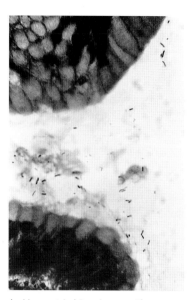

Fig. 8.3 (A) Distinctive morphology of *H. pylori* in gastric biopsies – uniform, curved, wavy, closely associated with epithelial surface, and usually present in large numbers **(B)** Other, mixed bacterial flora is present in patients with hypochlorhydia (e.g. on proton pump inhibitors) and must be distinguished from *H. pylori*

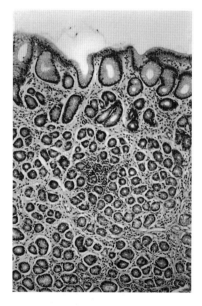

Fig. 8.4 Antral biopsy taken 2 years after eradication of *Helicobacter* gastritis.

over months and years (Fig. 8.4). It is not yet clear whether atrophy and intestinal metaplasia are reversible.

Within the spectrum of *Helicobacter* gastritis, topographical patterns can be recognized when biopsies (preferably two) from each site are taken. These include the following.

ANTRUM PREDOMINANT GASTRITIS

There is active chronic inflammation in the antrum, while the corpus mucosa shows only minimal or mild inflammation (Fig. 8.5), with *Helicobacter* present usually in smaller numbers in the corpus. Such patients have preserved or enhanced acid secretion, and this group includes patients with pyloric and duodenal ulcers. *Helicobacter* gastritis is associated with the disturbance in control of acid secretion long recognized in duodenal ulcer patients, and this is largely corrected by eradication of the organism.

SEVERE PAN GASTRITIS

Patients developing gastric ulcers in association with *H. pylori* tend to have a more severe gastritis, typically with prominent cytopathic changes of the surface epithelium. Neutrophils are present within the surface epithelium in addition to the more common location at the gastric pits (Fig. 8.6).[10,11] The rate of progression of atrophy, and frequency of intestinal metaplasia, is generally greater in *H. pylori* positive patients with a history of gastric ulcers, than in those without.

CORPUS PREDOMINANT GASTRITIS

A minority of patients (perhaps 5–10%) with *Helicobacter* have corpus predominant inflammation from an early stage. This interesting group appears to have hypochlorhydria well before the development of glandular atrophy and their acid production can therefore recover after eradication of *H. pylori*.[12] This pattern of gastritis is commoner among relatives of gastric cancer patients, and may represent a group at particular risk of developing gastric cancer, since their hypochlorhydria (known to be important in gastric carcinogenesis) is present from an early age.

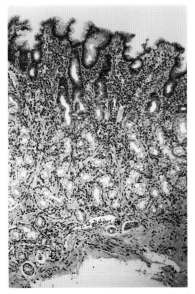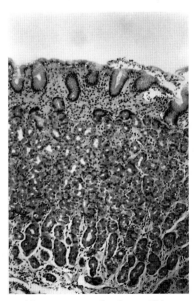

Fig. 8.5 (A) Antral; **(B)** corpus: *Helicobacter* gastritis, antrum predominant. This pattern of gastritis is associated with risk of duodenal or prepyloric ulceration.

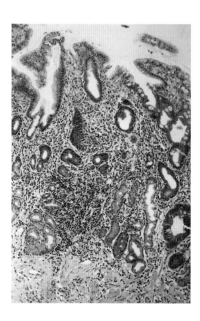

Fig. 8.6 Gastric corpus biopsy for a patient with gastric ulcer and *H. pylori*; there is atrophy, pyloric and intestinal metaplasia, and irregularity of surface epithelium.

HELICOBACTER AND GASTRIC CANCER

There are currently major changes in the epidemiology of gastric cancer.[13] Distal (i.e. non-cardia) cancer has been declining over the past few decades in most countries, while cardia adenocarcinoma, like adenocarcinoma of the distal oesophagus, has been increasing in Western countries. Non-cardia gastric cancers, both intestinal and diffuse types, are associated with *Helicobacter* gastritis, and their decline reflects the decreasing prevalence of *Helicobacter* gastritis in countries where socio-economic conditions have improved. The association of gastric cancer with current *Helicobacter* infection is strongest in younger patients,[14] in the elderly it is not apparent owing to two factors – the prevalence of *H. pylori* is higher in older people and *H. pylori* tends to disappear from the mucosa as atrophy and hypochlorhydria progress, so that by the time the cancer is diagnosed the infection is no longer present.

Gastric atrophy and intestinal metaplasia are commoner in patients with gastric cancer and in those populations with a high incidence of gastric cancer, and have been studied as potential markers of cancer risk strategies for screening for gastric cancer. Sulphomucin positive incomplete intestinal metaplasia (Type II b) has received most attention, but, at least in the UK, follow-up studies have not shown a high incidence of new cancers in patients with this type of intestinal metaplasia (IM).[15,16] Any IM is unusual in patients aged under 40 in the UK, but has been found in individuals with a strong family history of gastric cancer,[17] and eradication of *Helicobacter* is indicated in such patients.

GASTRIC MALT LYMPHOMA

Where the lymphocytic infiltrate is particularly dense, the question of gastric lymphoma arises. Low grade gastric MALT lymphoma is characterized by sheets of lymphocytes replacing gastric glands, and forming destructive lympho-epithelial lesions. These are usefully highlighted by cytokeratin stains (Fig. 8.7), which

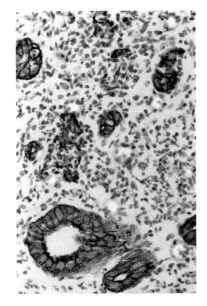

Fig. 8.7 Gastric biopsy from a patient with low grade gastric MALT lymphoma; immunostaining of cytokeratins (Cam 5.2) accentuates the destructive lymphoepithelial lesions.

may reveal additional lesions overlooked on the H & E.[18] Such lesions are also occasionally seen in severe chronic gastritis, and it may be difficult to make a firm diagnosis of low grade MALT lymphoma, unless molecular techniques to investigate clonality are available. The distinction is not essential for treatment since low grade lymphoma usually regresses after *Helicobacter* eradication therapy, but is important for follow-up, since relapse may occur despite *Helicobacter* eradication.[19]

H. HEILMANNII INFECTION

About 0.2% of endoscopied patients have gastric infections with the long spiral organism *H. heilmannii* (previously *Gastrospirillum*[20]), which does not generally infect patients with *H. pylori*. This causes a milder, inactive chronic gastritis, and the bacteria do not show the attachment to surface epithelium that is a characteristic of *H. pylori* (Fig. 8.8). Nevertheless, infections may sometimes be associated with duodenal ulceration. It is treated in the same way as *H. pylori*.

HELICOBACTER NEGATIVE GASTRITIS

Some patients have an increase in mononuclear cells in the gastric mucosa without *Helicobacter*. Possible explanations for this are listed in Table 8.1 and several have distinctive morphology, and are categorized as 'special forms' on the Sydney system.[2,3] Full classification requires clinicopathological correlation.

PREVIOUS OR SUPPRESSED H. PYLORI INFECTION

A pattern suggestive of *Helicobacter* gastritis, but without neutrophils, surface epithelial changes, or the bacteria, is likely to be due to previous infection. In particular, proton pump inhibitors, which suppress *H. pylori*, have often been used prior to endoscopy. This results in biopsies showing inactive, *H. pylori* negative

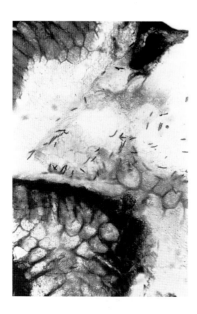

Fig. 8.8 *H. heilmannii* – a long corkscrew shaped bacterium that does not show the close association with surface epithelium characteristic of *H. pylori*.

Table 8.1 Differential diagnosis for Helicobacter negative gastritis

Previous or suppressed *Helicobacter* infection
Autoimmune gastritis

Special forms of gastritis:
 Reactive/chemical/reflux gastritis
 Lymphocytic gastritis
 Granulomatous gastritis
 Eosinophilic gastritis
 Rare infections e.g. CMV, *Giardia*.

gastritis, except in the proximal corpus where bacterial growth and inflammation may be enhanced.[21] H_2 receptor antagonists have a much less suppressive effect and *H. pylori* can usually still be seen in biopsies from patients treated with these agents. Most antibiotics suppress *H. pylori*, although when used singly for other infections they rarely eradicate *H. pylori*.

Previous *Helicobacter* infection can be detected by serology for up to several years, but alternative tests based on the presence of bacteria (i.e. biopsy urease (CLO) test, microbiological culture or urea breath test) will, like histology, be unreliable in patients with low bacterial load. Current treatment of *Helicobacter* gastritis is usually with 'triple therapy' (proton pump inhibitor plus two antibiotics for 1–2 weeks): with good patient compliance, this has an eradication rate of around 90%. Clinical indications for treating *Helicobacter* gastritis continue to be debated; some recommend treatment for those with more severe gastric pathology[22] implying the need for gastric biopsy before treatment, but increasingly the trend is for all infected patients to be treated.

AUTOIMMUNE GASTRITIS

Helicobacter negative corpus predominant gastritis with atrophy and intestinal metaplasia of the corpus mucosa, and near-normal antrum, is characteristic of autoimmune chronic gastritis,[23] (Fig. 8.9). Such patients will have achlorhydria,

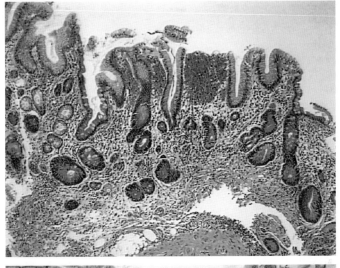

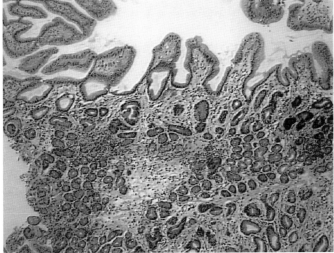

Fig. 8.9 Antrum **(A)** and corpus **(B)** biopsies from a patient with autoimmune gastritis – there is severe atrophy and intestinal metaplasia in corpus mucosa, while the antrum shows only mild atrophy.

and if they also have intrinsic factor autoantibodies, may have pernicious anaemia.[24] There is evidence that this condition may be triggered by *H. pylori* in susceptible individuals, since many are seropositive for *H. pylori*. However, by the time the condition is recognized, *H. pylori* (which is dependent on some gastric acid secretion) is usually not present. Neuroendocrine cell hyperplasia is commonly present in corpus biopsies from these patients, and may form 'microcarcinoid' tumours, but it is exceptionally rare for these tumours to metastasize, unless of a size greater than 2 cm.

TRUE *H. PYLORI* NEGATIVE GASTRITIS

CHEMICAL OR REACTIVE GASTRITIS

A common pattern of gastric mucosal injury characterized by foveolar hyperplasia (increased length and tortuosity of foveolae, with mucin depletion), oedema, congestion and (relative) lack of inflammatory cell infiltration is seen in patients following partial gastrectomy, where it is known as 'reflux gastritis'.[25] Similar, although usually milder, features are seen in patients without previous gastric surgery and the term 'chemical gastritis'[3] or 'reactive gastritis'[2] is used for this condition (Fig. 8.10).[26] In over half of these patients, a recognized cause of 'chemical' injury to the stomach (Non-Steroidal Anti-Inflammatory Drugs (NSAIDs), bile reflux, perhaps alcohol) can be identified, and portal hypertensive gastropathy gives a similar appearance in *Helicobacter* negative patients. In some patients, biopsies show features of both reactive gastritis (most notably foveolar hyperplasia) and *H. pylori* gastritis – unsurprising, since both are common disorders, and there is some synergy between them in gastric ulcerogenesis.

LYMPHOCYTIC GASTRITIS

The defining feature of this is the large number of intraepithelial lymphocytes – normally very sparse in gastric mucosa (3/100 surface epithelial cells). Counts of >25 intraepithelial lymphocytes per 100 surface epithelial cells identify lymphocytic gastritis (Fig. 8.11).[27] Patients with more severe involvement of the antral mucosa are likely to have coeliac disease, and should be further investigated for this.[28] Patients with predominantly corpus involvement are usually *H. pylori* positive serologically, although organisms may be very sparse and therefore not seen on biopsies. Whether or not *H. pylori* is seen on histology, these patients respond to the standard triple therapy treatment for *Helicobacter*.[29] Lymphocytic gastritis seems to be associated with hypochlorhydria and a rapid progression to corpus atrophy, and shows an association with gastric adenocarcinoma and lymphoma.[30]

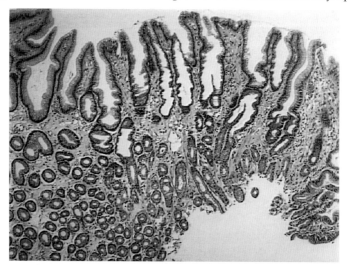

Fig. 8.10 Antral mucosa of a patient taking NSAIDs, showing foveolar hyperplasia with characteristic serrated pattern, but no increase in lamina propria cellularity. Oedema is frequently present although not in this example.

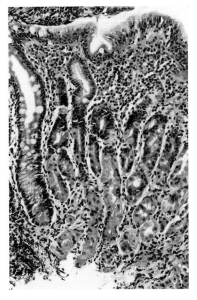

Fig. 8.11 Lymphocytic gastritis, in this case of the corpus mucosa, associated with atrophy and intestinal metaplasia.

GRANULOMATOUS GASTRITIS

Mucosal granulomas may be found in patients with or without *H. pylori*, and in *H. pylori* negative patients may be associated with Crohn's disease, sarcoidosis (Fig. 8.12) or represent idiopathic granulomatous gastritis where granulomas are often more numerous. Foreign body type granulomas can be seen in areas of previous mucosal erosion.

Crohn's disease is characterized by patchy, *Helicobacter* negative active gastritis with some areas of normal mucosa. Granulomas are sparse, and if Crohn's disease is suspected, it is worth searching for granulomas in multiple levels. Most patients have evidence of Crohn's disease at other sites, or endoscopic features suggesting Crohn's disease.

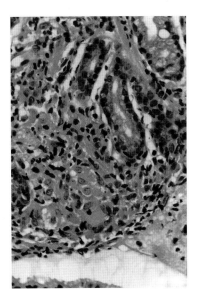

Fig. 8.12 Granulomatous gastritis – this patient had sarcoidosis.

RARE TYPES OF GASTRITIS

Other specific patterns of gastritis very rarely seen include eosinophilic gastritis (Fig. 8.13), cytomegalovirus (CMV) gastritis in immunocompromised individuals (Fig. 8.14), and *Giardia* in the stomach, in patients with hypochlorhydria and duodenal giardia. Features of reactive gastritis together with mucosal capillary microthrombi suggest gastric antral vascular ectasia (Watermelon stomach).[31] Menetrier's disease should be considered where foveolar hyperplasia is extreme – both diagnoses are associated with characteristic endoscopic appearances. Each of these are rare, seen in <0.5% of routine gastric biopsies.

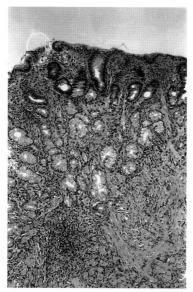 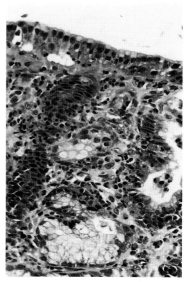

Fig. 8.13 Eosinophilic gastritis: **(A)** original magnification × 32 shows the transmucosal distribution of inflammation and associated fibrosis; **(B)** original magnification × 128 to show predominance of eosinophils in lamina propria and epithelium.

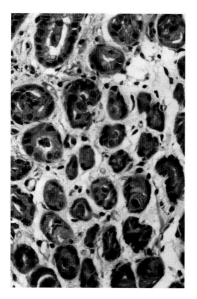

Fig. 8.14 Gastric biopsy from an immunosuppressed patient to show CMV inclusions, in this case in glandular epithelium, but endothelial cells and stromal cells may also show inclusions and the degree of associated inflammation is very variable.

USE OF GASTRIC BIOPSY

An audit of the use of gastric biopsies in 11 different hospitals in Yorkshire revealed that the proportion of endoscopies that included gastric biopsy varied from 10–94%.[32] This reflects a variation in policy between endoscopists ranging from those who use targeted biopsy of focal mucosal lesions to those who value knowledge of the histological state of the gastric mucosa. There is as yet no clinical consensus on this point. From a practical point of view it is important for the pathologist to be told whether a biopsy is a targeted one from a focal mucosal lesion or is intended to sample the 'background' gastric mucosa. In an audit of 9000 gastric biopsy requests in a centre with a high biopsy rate, neoplasia was diagnosed in 1.5% of patients and always in targeted biopsies or patients with previous evidence of dysplasia or malignancy.[33] Conversely, even when biopsies are restricted to focal lesions, the great majority will show features of one of the non-neoplastic conditions described above.

KEY POINTS

1. Gastric biopsies are among the most frequent specimens we receive.
2. Recognition of the particular characteristics of gastritis often gives clinically valuable information guiding diagnosis and treatment. When the pathologist receives clinical information including indication for endoscopy, endoscopic findings and details of recent medication, a clinicopathologically relevant report more informative than non-specific chronic gastritis can be given in the great majority of cases.
3. *Helicobactor pylori* has a high prevalence and involvement in nearly all gastric pathology.
4. Within the spectrum of *Helicobactor gastritis*, topographical patterns can be recognized, and six such patterns were described.
5. Various topographical patterns can be seen in *Helicobacter*–negative gastritis. These were also described and discussed.

REFERENCES

1. Marshall BJ, Warren JR. Unidentified curved bacilli on gastric epithelium in active chronic gastritis. Lancet 1983; i: 1273–1275
2. Price A B. The Sydney system: histological division. J Gastroenterol Hepatol 1991; 6: 209–222
3. Dixon MF, Genta RM, Yardley JH, Correa P. Classification and grading of gastritis: the upgraded Sydney system. Am J Surg Pathol 1996; 20: 1161–1181
4. Sternberg SS (Ed.). Histology for Pathologists, 2nd edn. New York: Lippincott-Raven, 1997. See Owen DA, Stomach pp. 483–487
5. Anderson JR (Ed.). Muir's Textbook of Pathology, 12th edn. London: Edward Arnold, 1985. See Lee FD, Alimentary tract, section III, Stomach pp 19.19
6 Lee A. Spiral organisms: what are they? A microbiological introduction to *Helicobacter pylori*. Scand J Gastroenterol 1991; 187 (suppl.): 9–22
7. Sobala GM, Crabtree JE, Dixon MF et al. Acute *Helicobacter pylori* infection: clinical features, local and systemic immune response, gastric mucosal histology and gastric juice ascorbic acid concentrations. Gut 1991; 32: 1415–1418

8. Gray SF, Wyatt JI, Rathbone BJ. Simplified techniques for identifying *Campylobacter pyloridis*. J Clin Pathol 1986; 39: 1279–1280

9. Genta RM, Robason GO, Graham DY. Simultaneous visualization of *Helicobacter pylori* and gastric morphology: a new stain. Hum Pathol 1994; 25: 221–226

10. Maaroos H-I, Kekki M, Sipponen P et al. Grade of *Helicobacter pylori* colonisation, chronic gastritis and relative risks of contracting high gastric ulcers; a seven year follow up. Scand J Gastroenterol 1991; 26 (suppl. 186): 65–72

11. Chan WY, Hui PK, Chan JKC et al. Epithelial damage by *Helicobacter pylori* in gastric ulcers. Histopathology 1991; 19: 47–53

12. El-Omar EM, Oien K, El-Nujumi A et al. *Helicobacter pylori* infection and chronic gastric acid hyposecretion. Gastroenterology 1997; 113: 15–24

13. Devesa SS, Blot WJ, Fraumeni JF Jr. Changing patterns in the incidence of esophageal and gastric carcinoma in the United States. Cancer 1998; 83: 2049–2053

14. Huang J-Q, Sridher S, Chen Y, Hunt R. Meta-analysis of the relationship between *Helicobacter pylori* seropositivity and gastric cancer. Gastroenterology 1998; 114: 1169–1179

15. Ectors N, Dixon MF. The prognostic value of sulphomucin positive intestinal metaplasia in the development of gastric cancer. Histopathology 1986; 10: 1271–1277

16 Ramesar KCRB, Sanders DSA, Hopwood D. Limited value of type III intestinal metaplasia in predicting risk of gastric carcinoma. J Clin Pathol 1987; 40: 1287–1290

17. Scott N, Lansdown M, Diament R et al. *Helicobacter* gastritis and intestinal metaplasia in a gastric cancer family. Lancet 1990; 335: 728 (Letter)

18. Wotherspoon AC, Donglioni C, de Boni M, Spencer J, Isaacson PG. Antibiotic treatment for low grade gastric MALT lymphoma. Lancet 1994; 343: 1503 (Letter)

19. Neubauer A, Thiede C, Morgner A et al. Cure of *Helicobacter pylori* infection and duration of remission of low-grade gastric mucosa-associated lymphoid tissue lymphoma. J Natl Cancer Inst 1997; 89: 1350–1355

20. Heilmann KL, Borchard F. Gastritis due to spiral shaped bacteria other than *Helicobacter pylori*: clinical, histological and ultra-structural findings. Gut 1991; 32: 137–140

21. Logan RP, Walker MM, Misiewicz JJ et al. Changes in the intragastric distribution of *Helicobacter pylori* during treatment with omeprazole. Gut 1995; 36: 12–16

22. Current European concepts in the management of *Helicobacter pylori* infection. The Masstricht Consensus Report. European *Helicobacter pylori* Study Group. Gut 1997; 41: 8–13

23. Flejou PF, Bahame P, Smith A et al. Pernicious anaemia and *Campylobacter*-like organisms: is the gastric antrum resistant to colonisation? Gut 1989; 30: 60–64

24. Burman P, Mardh S, Norberg L et al. Parietal cell antibodies in pernicious anaemia inhibit H^+, K^+ - adenosine triphosphatase, the proton pump of the stomach. Gastroenterology 1989; 96: 1434–1438

25. Dixon MF, O'Connor HJ, Axon ATR et al. Reflux gastritis: distinct histopathological entity? J Clin Pathol 1986; 39: 524–530

26. Sobah GM, King RFG, Axon ATR, Dixon MF. Reflux gastritis in the intact stomach. J Clin Pathol 1990; 43: 303–306

27. Dixon MF, Wyatt JI, Burke DA et al. Lymphocytic gastritis – relationship to *Campylobacter pylori* infection. J Pathol 1988; 154: 125–132

28. Hayat M, Arora DS, Wyatt JI, O'Mahoney S, Dixon MF. The pattern of involvement of the gastric mucosa in lymphocytic gastritis is predictive of the presence of duodenal pathology. J Clin Pathol 1999; 52: 815–819

29. Hayat M, Arora DS, Dixon MF, Clark B, O'Mahony S. Effects of *Helicobacter pylori* eradication on the natural history of lymphocytic gastritis. Gut 1999; 45: 495–498

30. Griffiths AP, Wyatt JI, Jack AS, Dixon MF. Lymphocytic gastritis, gastric adenocarcinoma and primary gastric lymphoma. J Clin Pathol 1994; 47: 1123–1124

31. Suit PF, Petras RD, Bauer TW, Petrini JL. Gastric antral vascular ectasia. A histologic and morphometric study of 'the watermelon stomach'. Am J Surg Pathol 1987; 11: 750–757

32. Sleight J, Wyatt JI. Variation in routine use of gastric biopsy histology. Unpublished report for the Yorkshire Audit

33. Cadman B, Dixon MF, Wyatt JI. Value of routine, non-targeted biopsies in the diagnosis of gastric neoplasia. J Clin Pathol 1997; 50: 832–834

9

Arterial remodelling: mechanisms of altered artery structure and their diagnostic implications for pathologists

G.B.M. Lindop   J. J. Boyle

INTRODUCTION

Blood vessels alter their geometry rapidly and reversibly in response to neuro-humoral stimuli and to tissue metabolites that signal altered functional demand. These rapid and reversible responses are investigated by physiologists and pharmacologists. However, sustained alteration in pressure and/or flow and the response to injury invariably lead to structural changes in blood vessels that then enter the domain of histopathologists. The term 'remodelling' was originally used to describe altered arterial geometry that was achieved by the rearrangement of existing smooth muscle cells. Unfortunately, because of the confusing vocabulary used to describe them, this term is now applied to almost any structural change in blood vessels.

> *When I use a word, it means exactly what I choose it to mean – neither more nor less (Humpty Dumpty, from Alice Through the Looking Glass, Lewis Carroll).*

Histological appearances can only be interpreted by understanding the physiological mechanisms involved. This chapter attempts to clarify for pathologists how arteries change their structure in response to altered flow and pressure, and then to consider how they repair themselves following damage.

STRUCTURE OF ARTERIES

Arteries consist of three coats: the intima, media and adventitia and all of them may be altered in disease. The normal intima consists of little more than a layer of endothelium that is permeable to small vasoactive molecules and selectively

G.B.M Lindop BSc, MB ChB, FRCP, FRCPath, Reader in Pathology, University of Glasgow Department of Pathology, Western Infirmary, Glasgow G11 6NT, UK

J.J. Boyle BSc, MB ChB, MRCPath MRC Clinical Training Fellow, Departments of Histopathology and Medicine, Addenbrooke's Hospital, Hills Road, Cambridge, CB2 2QQ, UK

permeable to macromolecules.[1] The intima is separated from the media by the internal elastic lamina. This cylinder of elastin is traditionally believed to resist the distending force of the blood pressure. However, since small veins contract more than arteries, to the point of obliteration of the lumen, the internal elastic lamina may also help to prevent complete vasoconstriction in small arteries, and hence potentially catastrophic ischaemia. The media consists of 'circular' smooth muscle – a tight spiral of spindle-shaped smooth muscle cells. The spindle shape of vascular smooth muscle cells and their spiral orientation means that the artery tends to lengthen both on medial smooth muscle contraction and on relaxation. The proportion of connective tissue matrix varies with the size of the artery, with the tissue supplied and with age.[2] The adventitia is a thin layer of loose connective tissue and contains mast cells, the lymphatics and the nerves that control vascular tone.[3]

THE CENTRAL ROLE OF THE ENDOTHELIUM

In early embryonic mesenchyme, endothelial cells are the first vascular cells to differentiate round spaces ('blood lakes'), which are the progenitors of blood vessels. It is likely that the endothelial cells regulate the growth, proliferation and differentiation of the other cell types in the developing blood vessel wall.[4] Although heterogeneous, mature endothelium is an active tissue. The endothelial cell secretes more than 30 known regulatory molecules.[5] Endothelial function is not only crucial in vasomotion – endothelial dependent relaxation and constriction (see below), but the endothelium also controls haemostasis by modulating platelet activation, coagulation and fibrinolysis.[5,6] The endothelium also regulates the permeability of the circulation and hence the access of circulating regulatory molecules to tissue cells and to other cells in the vessel wall.[1] Figure 9.1 illustrates these interactions with the blood and depicts the key role of the endothelial cell in determining the differentiation of new vessels (angiogenesis) and the response of mature arteries to physiological stimuli and to damage.

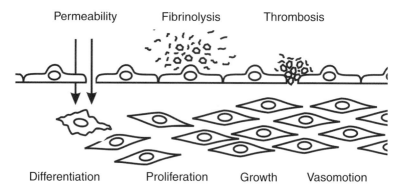

Fig. 9.1 The endothelium modulates permeability and therefore the egress of circulating molecules. The endothelium also interacts with the blood by controlling haemostasis by the expression of pro-thrombotic and anti-thrombotic molecules on its surface. In addition, many endothelial regulatory molecules influence vasomotion in the short term and, in the long term, growth, proliferation, migration and differentiation of the smooth muscle cells in the artery wall.

INTERACTIONS BETWEEN VASOMOTION, THROMBOSIS, FIBRINOLYSIS AND CELL GROWTH

VASOMOTION AND GROWTH – THE AMPLIFIERS

Vasoconstrictors raise blood pressure and thereby increase wall tension and medial smooth muscle workload. If sustained, as in hypertension, medial hypertrophy ensues. However, vasoconstrictors also stimulate growth by a direct action on cells: for example, angiotensin II stimulates the growth of most cultured cells; likewise, other potent vasoconstrictors such as catecholamines and endothelins also stimulate growth.[7-9] Furthermore, recombinant platelet derived growth factor (PDGF), the most important circulating growth factor [10,11] is a powerful vasoconstrictor.[12]

Conversely, vasodilators such as nitric oxide and prostacyclin inhibit cell growth.[5,9] In addition to direct inhibition of cell growth, vasodilatators reduce cell growth indirectly by lowering blood pressure, wall tension and medial workload. The duality of vasoactive agents that affect growth and vasomotion in the context of hypertension has recently been dubbed the 'humoral amplifier'.[13]

In early hypertension, medial thickening and a larger wall-to-lumen ratio increase the force of contraction for a given size of artery. This change in the geometry of blood vessels became known as the 'vascular amplifier'.[7,14] Thus in early hypertension, vascular and humoral amplifiers may act in concert to promote medial thickening.

THROMBOSIS AND GROWTH

The endothelium regulates haemostasis by actions on the activities of platelets and the clotting system, by the secretion of regulatory molecules and by the expression of pro-coagulant and anti-coagulant molecules on its luminal surface: for example, prostacyclin and nitric oxide are platelet inhibitors,[5] whereas thrombin and thromboxane secreted by platelets are pro-coagulants and vasoconstrictors.[15-17] Vasodilators are usually anti-coagulants and inhibit cell growth while vasoconstrictors tend to be pro-coagulant and stimulate cell growth. In an injured artery, vasoconstriction and thrombosis act together to prevent haemorrhage; then, increased cell growth and proliferation act to organize thrombus and to repair damage.

FIBRINOLYSIS AND GROWTH

Recently, a novel peptide, angiostatin, derived from the plasmin molecule has been found to strongly inhibit endothelial cell proliferation.[18] When fibrinolysis is activated along with thrombosis, angiostatin, derived from the proteolysis of plasmin, could act as a negative counterbalance to the growth stimulating effect of thrombosis following damage to the vessel wall. The potential interplay between vasomotion haemostasis and their probable effect on cell growth in blood vessels is summarized in Fig. 9.2.

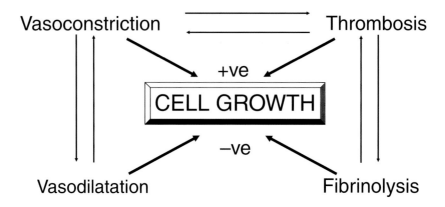

Fig. 9.2 This illustrates the potential in vivo interactions between the molecules that regulate vasomotion and haemostasis and their probable effects on cell growth.

MEDIATORS OF ALTERED ARTERIAL STRUCTURE

The main physiological stimuli affecting artery structure are neurohumoral influences and physical forces generated by the flow and pressure of the blood.

NEUROHUMORAL INFLUENCES

These circulate in the blood and are released from platelets, nerves and other cells in the artery wall. In systemic arteries, unlike veins and pulmonary arteries, only the outer layer of smooth muscle cells are innervated and depolarization is transmitted to all of the smooth muscle cells via cell junctions.[3] Circulating vasoactive agents influence vascular tone by two pathways: a direct effect on the medial smooth muscle after passing through the endothelium, and a separate action on the endothelium to modulate the release of endothelial derived vasoactive agents, which affect smooth muscle cell function. The overall neurohumoral control of arteries is therefore mediated by the interplay of neurotransmitters released from nerves on their outer aspect, circulating molecules that pass through the endothelium and other mediators secreted by the endothelium and by the smooth muscle cells themselves. Some of the most important molecules secreted by the various arterial cell types and their probable effect on artery growth are listed in Table 9.1.

PHYSICAL FORCES

In addition to the fine control exerted by neurohumoral stimuli, blood vessels respond to physical forces generated by the flow of blood; this area has been recently reviewed.[27] The most important forces are wall tension (the distending force of the blood pressure), and shear stress (the frictional force of flowing blood). These forces may affect all layers of the vessel wall, but shear stress affects mainly the endothelium and wall tension affects principally the media.

Table 9.1 Some mediators of arterial remodelling

Endothelium		Smooth muscle		Nerves	
Mediator	*Growth*	*Mediator*	*Growth*	*Mediator*	*Growth*
Endothelin	+	PDGF	+	NA	+
13-HODE	+	IGF-1	+	NPY	+
FGF	+	FGF	+	FGF	+
PDGF	+	EGF	+	IL-1/PDGF	+
ACE/Ang II	+	IL-1	+/–	HGF	+
?BK	+	TGF	+/–	NGF	+
HETEs	+	TNF-α	+/–	ATP	+/–
Nitric oxide	–	Nitric oxide	–	Substance P	+/–
PGI2	–	GAG	–	CGRP	+/–
Heparinoids	–			VIP	–

13-HODE = 13-hydroxy-9, 11-octadecadienoic acid; FGF = fibroblast growth factor; PDGF = platelet derived growth factor; ACE = angiotensin converting enzyme; Ang II = angiotensin ii; BK = bradykinin; HETE = hydroxyeicosatetraenoic acid; PGI2 = prostacyclin; IGF-1 = insulin-like growth factor-1; EGF = epidermal growth factor; IL-1 = interleukin-1; TGF = Transforming growth factor; TNF-α = tumour necrosis factor-α; GAG = glycosaminoglycans; NA = noradrenaline; NPY = neuropeptide–Y; HGF = hepatocyte growth factor; NGF = nerve growth factor; ATP = adenosine triphosphate; CRGP = calcitonin gene-related peptide.

Sources: see references 5, 9–11, 19–27.

INCREASED FLOW

Both conduit and muscular arteries dilate to accommodate increased flow.[28,29] A rise in shear stress causes the endothelium to release vasodilators such as prostacyclin and nitric oxide and to decrease synthesis of vasoconstrictors such as endothelin.[21] The precise operation of the cellular transducers are not clear, but increased shear stress acts on the cytoskeleton, cell junctions and also opens ion channels in the endothelial cell membrane. The best characterized are K+ channels[28] but calcium channels are probably also involved as intracellular calcium increases.[8] Numerous second messenger systems and transcription factors are also activated (see Gimbrone[25]) and these also modulate the secretion of endothelial mediators; the most important effect is probably increasing the generation of nitric oxide (NO) and prostacyclin.

The resulting vasodilatation makes the media thinner; and, if pressure remains constant, increases wall tension per unit area, by simple physics (Laplace's law). If sustained, this increased work leads to hypertrophy of medial smooth muscle in the dilated vessel.[7,14] This is augmented by trophic factors; for example secretion of PDGF-B is regulated by shear stress response elements within the promoter sequence of its gene.[30]

How endothelial and medial smooth muscle cells grow, and are rearranged round a larger lumen is uncertain, but the outcome is overall enlargement of the vessel (Fig. 9.3). In the long term, the vessel usually elongates and becomes tortuous.

DECREASED FLOW

The endothelium senses falling shear stress; it decreases the synthesis of vasodilators such as prostacyclin and nitric oxide and increases the output of vasoconstrictors such as endothelin.[31] Because vasoconstrictors also stimulate cell growth,

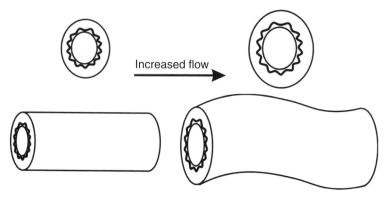

Fig. 9.3 Increased flow raises the shear stress on the endothelium, which releases vasodilators. Iinitially this causes vasodilatation which, in turn, leads ultimately to medial growth and overall enlargement of the artery without intimal proliferation.

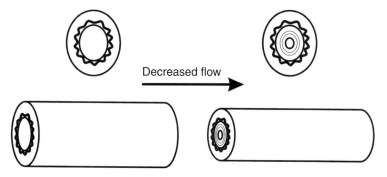

Fig. 9.4 Decreased flow lowers shear stress and increases endothelial synthesis of vasoconstrictors/growth promoters that initially cause vasoconstriction and eventually intimal proliferation.

the haemodynamic changes eventually lead to proliferation and migration of smooth muscle cells in the underlying media. Medial smooth muscle cells then migrate through into the intima where they orientate themselves circumferentially and lay down matrix. Intimal proliferation narrows the artery and thereby restores endothelial shear stress to normal by reduced flow through a narrower lumen. The reduction in wall tension per unit area and medial workload leads to atrophy, which is accompanied by increased smooth muscle cell apoptosis.[32] Obliteration of the lumen may be accelerated by thrombosis, which tends to complicate any stenosis. This is the mechanism of arterial involution: it is depicted in Fig. 9.4 and is discussed further below.

ALTERED PRESSURE

Hypertension increases wall tension and medial workload. This causes medial thickening to increase and consequently increases the wall/lumen ratio.[7,14,33] The roles of remodelling in the strict sense (increased wall/lumen ratio by rearrangement of the same number of medial smooth muscle cells round a smaller lumen), smooth muscle cell hyperplasia and hypertrophy have been extensively debated.[33,34] In humans, the relative contributions of remodelling and smooth

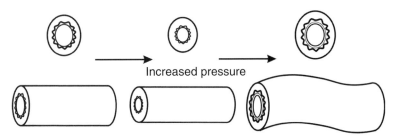

Fig. 9.5 Hypertension initially causes remodelling of the same number of smooth muscle cells around a smaller lumen, it then causes medial hypertrophy. In the long term, increased matrix synthesis causes stretching of the artery which becomes tortuous and shows secondary intimal proliferation.

muscle cell growth may vary with the aetiology of the hypertension.[35] Activation of the renin–angiotensin system has been implicated in promoting growth in hypertension and, conversely, treatment with inhibitors of this system may be more effective in lowering arterial wall/lumen ratio than other anti-hypertensive agents.[36,37]

Long-standing medial hypertrophy is accompanied by increased synthesis of matrix proteins giving rise to arteriosclerosis. Significant increase in matrix is followed by muscle atrophy in the media.[2] As muscle is replaced by matrix the arterial tree stretches. Elongation leads to tortuosity and dilatation causes a fall in shear stress that is counteracted by intimal proliferation, which restores the shear stress to normal (Fig. 9.5).

INJURY

All three layers of the artery may be injured separately or together. *Endothelial* injury varies in severity. Mild injury causes endothelial cell contraction, which opens intercellular gaps. In arteries, the earliest visible effect may be oedema of the intima.[38] Increased endothelial permeability causes plasma proteins to flood into the walls of small arteries and arterioles.[39] They accumulate initially as lozenge-shaped deposits in the intima, then the medial smooth muscle becomes replaced by proteinaceous deposits.[2] This process has been called 'plasmatic vasculosis', a term that has never become popular but for which there is no substitute. In acute plasmatic vasculosis, the artery wall is saturated with homogeneous protein material with the staining reactions of fibrin. Some authors have used the term 'fibrinoid necrosis' for this appearance; however, it seems sensible to reserve the use of the term 'necrosis' for lesions with histological evidence of cellular necrosis or apoptosis.[13]

More severe injuries cause endothelial denudation. Experimental balloon injury has been extensively studied. Exposed collagen in the underlying artery wall usually causes monocyte and platelet adhesion with thrombosis and release of growth promoting factors such as PDGF.[11] After lysis of thrombus, endothelial cell division and migration repair the defect, within a few hours if small. Chronic injury or healing of more severe acute injury leads to intimal proliferation. Intimal thickening again lowers mean wall tension and leads to atrophy of the overlying media; this is discussed further below.

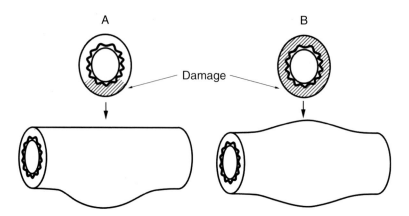

Fig. 9.6 Segmental medial damage (hatched area) causes weakening which leads to a saccular aneurysm (**A**) while circumferential damage causes a fusiform aneurysm (**B**).

The syndrome of 'endothelial dysfunction' is associated with an imbalance in the secretion of vasodilator/vasoconstrictor molecules. This is common in hypertension, diabetes and hyperlipidaemia.[40] There are no morphological stigmata, but low-grade endothelial injury could be inferred. In atherogenesis, candidate causes of chronic endothelial injury include oxidized low density lipid (LDL), hyperhomocysteinaemia and perhaps chemicals derived from cigarette smoke.

Medial injury due to trauma may cause fibrosis and disturbance of the smooth muscle cell architecture.[41] Weakening of the artery wall may cause dilatation. Segmental weakening causes a saccular aneurysm (Fig. 9.6A) and circumferential weakening leads to a fusiform aneurysm (Fig. 9.6B). In the aneurysm, intimal proliferation and thrombosis are promoted by a fall in endothelial shear stress and turbulence due to dilatation. Thrombosis is probably also involved but its relative contribution is uncertain.

The adventitia is exposed to increased wall tension as a result of medial weakening and it responds with thickening and fibrosis.[41] It also undergoes scarring from direct injury. This is especially prominent in those types of vasculitis that destroy the media.

The response of arteries to all insults is best viewed as a modified form of healing – similar in essential respects to wound healing elsewhere. The 'response to injury' hypothesis of atherogenesis was proposed to emphasize the fact that similar cellular events may occur in the early plaque. However, the response to angioplasty is the best studied experimental model of artery injury[42] and is the main setting in which some of the processes discussed below have been elucidated.

CELLULAR RESPONSES TO INJURY

Severe endothelial injury or loss affects all layers of the vessel wall. First, fibrin and platelets adhere to exposed collagen in the denuded wall. Formation of thrombin and the release of 5-hydroxytryptamine and thromboxane from platelets cause vasoconstriction. Platelets also release the cytokines PDGF and transforming growth factor beta (TGF-β), which stimulate smooth vascular smooth muscle cell migration and collagen synthesis, respectively. Medial smooth muscle cells change from their contractile phenotype into so-called 'synthetic' vascular smooth muscle cells that are indistinguishable from myofibroblasts.[43] As in wounds, synthetic smooth muscle cells migrate to the injury, where they divide and lay down matrix. Eventually they are lost by apoptosis.[44] Endothelial cells also divide and migrate, as in wound angiogenesis: they cover surface defects in damaged arteries and form new vessels in organizing thrombus and in atheromatous plaques; however both angiogenesis and atherogenesis are beyond the scope of this chapter.

CONTROL OF MIGRATION, PROLIFERATION, APOPTOSIS AND MATRIX PRODUCTION

Migration of arterial vascular smooth muscle cells is a complex process; it involves digestion of matrix by metalloproteinase enzymes and then actin/myosin interactions to bring about cell motility[45] in order to respond to chemotactic concentration gradients. PDGF seems to be the main regulator of vascular smooth muscle cell migration in vivo.[45] Other candidates include complement and fibrin degradation products.[46] The capacity of cells to sense a PDGF concentration gradient seems to be linked to activation of the novel second messenger Phosphatidyl Inositol-3-hyroxl-kinase (Pt-3-OH kinase).[47]

Proliferation of vascular smooth muscle cells is stimulated by innumerable mitogens among which PDGF, fibroblast growth factor (FGF) and Angiotensin II (AII) seem to be the strongest candidates.[8,9] Importantly, PDGF mediates mitogenesis induced by the pro-inflammatory cytokine interleukin-1 (IL-1).[48] This connection makes PDGF a potentially important mediator of the link between local inflammation and the resulting intimal proliferation. At the transcriptional factor level, most growth factors stimulate mitogen activated protein kinase (MAPK) and elevate Activating protein (AP)-1, whereas most pro-inflammatory stimuli activate Nuclear-factor-kappaB (NF-kB). However, there is cross-talk between AP-1 and NF-kB transcriptional factors; thus inflammation and the proliferative response to injury are tightly linked at both the signal and transcriptional factor levels.[49–51]

Matrix synthesis is probably mediated largely by TGF-β, which is mitogenic only in some circumstances; in culture it mediates contact inhibition and inhibits mitosis in vascular smooth muscle cells. The most important action of TGF-β in vivo is to stimulate collagen and proteoglycan synthesis. TGF-β activates transcriptional factors, which bind directly to collagen gene promoters.[52,53]

Apoptosis follows intrinsic stimuli such as senescence or clonal exhaustion after rapid proliferation. In addition, metazoan cells probably undergo apoptosis without extrinsic stimuli such as 'survival signals' from other cells and matrix contact.[54] Matrix-derived signals are probably mediated by integrins.[55,56] Since vascular smooth muscle cells secrete matrix, they may also influence each other's survival via matrix/integrin interaction. Extrinsic stimuli include cytokines such as IL-1β, TNF-α, interferon-γ (IFN-γ) and NO.[57] The survival signals in vivo are uncertain but many candidates suggested by in vitro experiments include a number of known mitogens.

In addition to matrix-derived and extrinsic chemical signals, the haemodynamic forces of increased shear stress (flow) and stretch (blood pressure) activate specific vascular ion channels, MAPKinase and AP-1 signalling; correspondingly,

11. Ross R. Atherosclerosis – an inflammatory disease. N Engl J Med 1999, 340; 115–126

12. Berk BC, Alexander RW, Brock TA, Gimbrone MA Jr, Webb RC. Vasoconstriction: a new activity for platelet-derived growth factor. Science 1986; 232: 87–90

13. Lindop GBM, Jardine AG. Recent concepts and misconceptions in hypertension. In Kirkham N, Lemoine N (Eds) Progress in Pathology, volume 4. Edinburgh: Churchill Livingstone, 1997; 125–138

14. Folkow B. Physiological aspects of primary hypertension. Physiol Rev 1982, 62; 347–504

15. Wu KK, Thiagarajan P. Role of endothelium in thrombosis and hemostasis. Ann Rev Med 1996; 47: 315–331

16. Cines DB, Pollak ES, Buck CA et al. Endothelial cells in physiology and in the pathophysiology of vascular disorders. Blood 1998; 91; part 10; 3527–3561

17. Pearson JD, Vessel wall interactions regulating thrombosis. Brit Med Bull 1994; 50: 776–788

18. Clement B, Musso O, Lietard J, Theret N. Homeostatic control of angiogenesis: a newly identified function of the liver? Hepatology 1999; 29: 621–623

19. Langille BL. Remodelling of developing and mature arteries: endothelium, smooth muscle and matrix. J Cardiovasc Pharmacol 1993; 21 (suppl 1): S11–S17

20. Dzau VJ, Gibbons GH. Endothelium and growth factors in vascular remodeling of hypertension. Hypertension 1991; 18: III115–III121

21. Dzau VJ, Gibbons GH. Vascular remodelling: mechanisms and implications. J Cardiovasc Pharmacol 1993; 21 (suppl 1): S1–S5

22. Reidy MA, Fingerle J, Lindner V. Factors controlling the development of arterial lesions after injury. Circulation 1992; 86: III43–III46

23. Thyberg J, Hedin U, Sjolund M, Palmberg L, Bottger BA. Regulation of differentiated properties and proliferation of arterial smooth muscle cells. Arteriosclerosis 1990; 10: 966–990

24. Edvinsson L, Hakanson R, Wahlstadt C, Uddman R. Effects of neuropeptide-Y on the cardiovascular system. Trends Pharmacol Sci 1987; 8: 231–235

25. Gimbrone MA. Vascular endothelium, haemodynamic forces and atherogenesis. Am J Pathol 1999; 155: 1–5

26. Langille BL, O'Donnell F. Reductions in arterial diameter produced by chronic decreases in blood flow are endothelium-dependent. Science 1986; 231: 405–407

27. Resnick N, Gimbrone MA Jr. Haemodynamic forces – complex regulators of endothelial gene expression. Federation of Associations for Experimental Journal 1995; 9: 874–882

28. Cook JP, Rarsitch E, Andon NA, Lascalzo JJ, Dzau VJ. Flow activates an endothelial potassium channel to release an endogenous nitrovasodilator. J Clin Invest 1991, 88: 1663–1671

29. Koller A, Kaley G. Endothelial regulation of wall shear stress and blood flow in skeletal muscle microcirculation. Am J Physiol 1991; 260: H862–H868

30. Resnick N, Collins T, Atkinson W et al. Platelet-derived growth factor B chain promoter contains a cis-acting fluid shear-stress-response element. Proc Natl Acad Sci USA 1993; 90: 4591–4598

31. Anggard E. Nitric oxide: mediator, murderer and medicine. Lancet 1994, 343: 1199–1206

32. Cho A, Courtman DW, Langille BL. Apoptosis (programmed cell death) in arteries of the neonatal lamb. Circ Res 1995; 76: 168–175

33. Heagerty AM, Aalkjaer C, Bund SJ, Korsgaard N, Mulvaney MJ. Small artery structure in hypertension. Dual processes in remodelling and growth. Hypertension 1993; 21: 391–397

34. Mulvaney MJ. Resistance vessel structure in hypertension: growth or remodelling? J Cardiovasc Pharmacol 1993; 22 (suppl. 5): S44–S47

35. Rizzoni D, Porter E, Castellano M et al. Vascular hypertrophy and remodelling in secondary hypertension. Hypertension 1996; 28: 785–790

36. Thybo NK, Stephens N, Cooper A et al. Effects of anti-hypertensive treatment on small arteries of patients with previously untreated hypertension. Hypertension 1995; 25: 474–481

37. Schriffren EL. Correction of remodelling and function of small arteries in human hypertension by cilazapril, and angiotensin converting enzyme inhibitor. J Cardiovasc Pharmacol 1996; 27(suppl 2): S13–S18

38. Isles CG, McLay A, Jones JMB. Recovery in malignant hypertension presenting as acute renal failure. Q J Med 1984; 53: 439–452

39. Giese B. The Pathogenesis of Hypertensive Vascular Disease. Copenhagen: Muncksgaard, 1966
40. Wilkinson IB, Cockcroft JR. Cholesterol, endothelial function and cardiovascular disease. Curr Opin Lipidol 1998; 9: 237–242
41. Boyle JJ, Lawrie G, McPhaden AR, Richens D, Lindop GBM. Arterial lesions associated with remodelling in endomyocardial biopsies from human cardiac allografts. Histopathology 1995; 27: 439–444
42. Ferns GA, Raines EW, Sprugel KH et al. Inhibition of neointimal smooth muscle accumulation after angioplasty. Science 1991; 253: 1129–1132
43. Shi Y, O'Brian JE, Fard A et al. Adventitial myofibroblasts contribute to neointimal formation in injured porcine coronary arteries. Circulation 1996; 94: 1655–1664
44. Bochaton Piallat ML, Gabbiani F, Redard M, Desmouliere A, Gabbiani G. Apoptosis participates in cellularity regulation during rat aortic intimal thickening. Am J Pathol 1995; 146: 1059–1064
45. Newby AC, Zaltsman AB. Fibrous cap formation or destruction – the critical importance of vascular smooth muscle cell proliferation, migration and matrix formation. Cardiovasc Res 1999; 41: 345–360
46. Torzewski J, Bowyer DE, Waltenberger J, Fitzsimmons C. Processes in atherogenesis: complement activation. Atherosclerosis 1997; 132: 131–138
47. Kundra V, Escobedo JA, Kazlauskas A et al. Regulation of chemotaxis by the platelet-derived growth factor receptor-beta. Nature 1994; 367: 474–482
48. Raines EW, Dower SK, Ross R. Interleukin 1 mitogenic activity for fibroblasts and smooth muscle cells is due to PDGF-AA. Science 1989; 253: 393–396
49. Lindroos PM, Rice AB, Wang YZ, Bonner JC. Role of nuclear factor-κB and mitogen-activated protein kinase signaling pathways in IL-1 β-mediated induction of alpha-PDGF receptor expression in rat pulmonary myofibroblasts. J Immunol 1998; 161: 3464–3468
50. Schulze-Osthoff K, Ferrari D, Riehemann K, Wesselborg S. Regulation of NF-κB activation by MAP kinase cascades. Immunobiology 1997; 198: 35–49
51. Schwenzer R, Siemienski K, Liptay S et al. The human tumor necrosis factor (TNF) receptor-associated factor 1 gene (TRAF1) is up-regulated by cytokines of the TNF ligand family and modulates TNF-induced activation of NF-κB and c-Jun N-terminal kinase. J Biol Chem 1999; 274: 19368–19374
52. Suzuki S, Ebihara I, Tomino Y, Koide H. Transcriptional activation of matrix genes by transforming growth factor beta 1 in mesangial cells. Exp Nephrol 1993; 4: 229–237
53. Ritzenthaler JD, Goldstein RH, Fine A, Smith BD. Regulation of the alpha 1(I) collagen promoter via a transforming growth factor-beta activation element. J Biol Chem 1993; 268: 13625–13631
54. Raff MC. Size control: the regulation of cell numbers in animal development. Cell 1996; 86: 173–175
55. Giancotti FG, Ruoslahti E. Integrin signaling. Science 1999; 285: 1028–1032
56. Dejana E, Raiter M, Resnati M, Lampugnani MG. Endothelial integrins and their role in maintaining the integrity of the vessel wall. Kidney Int 1993; 43: 62–65
57. Geng YJ, Wu Q, Muszynski M, Hansson GK, Libby P. Apoptosis of vascular smooth muscle cells induced by in vitro stimulation with interferon-γ, tumour necrosis factor-α and interleukin-1β. Arterioscler Thromb Vasc Biol 1996; 16: 19–27
58. Courtman DW, Cho A, Langille L, Wilson GJ. Eliminating arterial pulsatile strain by external banding induces medial but not neointimal atrophy and apoptosis in the rabbit. Am J Pathol 1998; 153: 1723–1729
59. Davies MJ. Coronary artery remodelling and the assessment of stenosis by pathologists. Histopathology 1998; 33: 497–500
60. Peh SC, Lindop GBM. Chronic pyelonephritis: the significance of renal renin and the vascular changes in the human kidney. J Pathol 1991; 163: 343–349
61. Berry CL. Organogenesis of the arterial wall. In Camilleri J-P, Berry CL, Fiessinger J-N, Bariety J (Eds) Diseases of the Arterial Wall. Berlin: Springer Verlag, 1987; 55–68
62. Lindop GBM. Renovascular disease. In McGee J O'D, Isaacson PG, Wright NA (Eds) Oxford Textbook of Pathology. Oxford: Oxford University Press, 1992; 1470–1477

63. Lindop GBM. The renin-secreting cell in health and disease. In Robertson JIS, Nicholls MG (Eds) The Renin-Angiotensin System. London: Gower Medical Publishing, 1992; 19.1–19.15

64. Billingham ME. Histopathology of graft coronary disease. J Heart Lung Transplant 1992; 11: S38–44

65. Normann SJ, Salomon DR, Leelachaikul P et al. Acute vascular rejection of the coronary arteries in human heart transplantation: pathology and correlations with immunosuppression and cytomegalovirus infection. J Heart Lung Transplant 1991; 10: 674–687

66. Lindop GBM. The pulmonary circulation in left heart failure. In Peacock AJ (Ed.) The Pulmonary Circulation. A Handbook for Clinicians. London: Chapman & Hall, 1996; 245–242

67. Short D. Morphology of the intestinal arterioles in chronic human hypertension. Br Heart J 1966; 28: 184–192

68. Carr ND, Faragher EB, Hasleton PS. Quantitative study of intimal longitudinal smooth muscle in human small mesenteric arteries. Acta Anat (Basel) 1988; 132: 69–73

69. Glagov S. Intimal hyperplasia, vascular modeling and the restenosis problem. Circulation 1994; 89: 2888–2891

10

Error in histopathology

Suzanne L Wakely   Patrick J Gallagher

Histopathologists frequently disagree about microscopic diagnoses. Some of this disagreement is the result of undoubted difficulty in defining individual histological entities. A number of studies have shown that experienced, or even experienced and expert histopathologists, disagree in their interpretation of individual types of biopsy.[1-6] Some of these are in acknowledged areas of difficulty, such as malignant lymphoma or melanoma.[7-10] Everyday specimens such as cervical and gastric biopsies and uterine curettings can pose genuine difficulties, if not in diagnosis at least in grading. Notwithstanding this, there have been a number of publicized reports of error in histopathological diagnosis and, paradoxically, this has increased the profile of the surgical histopathologist.

There are now detailed requirements for quality control in cervical cytology and in England the Department of Health has instituted clear mechanisms to ensure that these are followed. As yet, there is no similar requirement for histopathology. This may well be introduced in the future and could be a requirement for laboratory accreditation. In this review we describe how and why pathologists make errors and the methods that are available to detect and prevent these.

HOW COMMON IS HISTOLOGICAL ERROR

All staff involved in health care pride themselves on the standard of their care and view error as an unfortunate event. This is particularly true in histopathology as a biopsy report is widely viewed as the definitive diagnostic procedure. All histopathologists make errors and some record them in their own, usually private, way! But how common are mistakes in routine practice? Our laboratory instituted a process of retrospective peer review 10 years ago and ran the system

Suzanne L. Wakely BM (Hons), MRCP, Specialist Registrar, Department of Radiology, Southampton University Hospitals, Southampton, SO16 6YD, UK

Patrick J. Gallagher MD, PhD, FRCPath, Reader, Consultant Histopathlogist, Southampton University Hospitals, Southampton, SO16 6YD, UK

They needed to measure information to ensure the coding systems were optimal. This was a practical spur to the study of information but a complete mathematical treatment was not produced until Shannon published his seminal work in 1948.[1] The development of the mathematical and physical basis of the digital computer by Turing and von Neumann also brought the concept of information to the forefront. Computers are essentially information processing systems. The Second World War provided an enormous boost to the study of information. Breaking the Enigma code, in which Turing played a major role, was one of the most important parts of the war effort. In fighting the war information was as important, and as real, as tanks, aeroplanes and bombs. It was shortly after the war, in 1948, that Shannon produced his mathematical theory of information, and shortly thereafter, in 1952, that Watson and Crick worked out the structure of DNA, the molecule of information (Table 11.1).

Watson and Crick realized that their model of DNA allowed sequential bases to act as a code, and the double helix could separate allowing self replication that would pass the information to the next generation. Crick burst into the Eagle Pub in Cambridge and announced, modestly, that they had found the secret of life. He told anybody who would listen that they had discovered how life begets life. Crick was in fact asserting that information was the basic concept in biology and that life could be understood in terms of the information contained in the DNA code. The revolution in molecular biology that has followed Watson and Crick's discovery is testimony to the importance of this assertion that information is fundamental.

In medicine the majority of us are now surrounded by the artefacts of the information age. All trainees in histopathology are expected to be familiar with digital computers and to use them for word processing, literature searches, e-mail communication and data storage. We are all expected to be familiar with molecular biology and its contribution to understanding biological function. The mathematical basis of the age of information and the work of Shannon, however, are not well known. I think this is unfortunate as the age of information is not just about using computers and telecommunication as tools. The concept of

Table 11.1 Milestones in the development of the concept of information

St John: 'In the beginning was the word, and the word was with God and the word was God.' – a succinct statement that creation is about information rather than energy.
Boltzmann: In 1894 Boltzmann remarked that energy is related to missing information – he realized that increased entropy is equivalent to reduced information.
Heisenberg: In 1927 Heisenberg established the uncertainty principle – this showed that the relationship between cause and effect is stochastic and changed the way we think about the physical universe.
Turing and von Neumann: In 1935 Turing and von Neumann met in Cambridge, UK. In the next decade they independently laid the mathematical and physical foundation of the digital computer.
Second World War: The breaking of the Enigma code, in which Turing played a major role, was of central importance in the war effort.
Shannon: In 1948 Shannon[1] established the mathematical theory of information.
Crick and Watson: In 1952 Crick and Watson worked out the structure of DNA, showed it was the molecule of information and ushered in the molecular biological revolution.

information, like the concept of energy in physics, can be used to develop a deeper understanding of biology and guide us in studying health and disease.

Information, energy and uncertainty are in fact closely related ideas. High energy chemical bonds are highly improbable structures that tend to break down to more probable structures. In the process energy is released and entropy increased. Improbable structures contain information and when they break down to more probable structures information is lost and uncertainty increases. An important problem in physics is how it is possible in the big bang to go from nothing to a large amount of energy in a fraction of a second when a central tenet of physics is that energy cannot be created nor destroyed. Information, however, can be created and destroyed, and information once created, can liberate energy. It is possible, therefore, that in the future information could become as important in physics as it will in biology.

GENERAL PRINCIPLES

Alan Turing, who played a major role in developing the digital computer, was primarily interested in understanding how the mind works. He wanted to show that the mind was a machine and he believed it should be possible to produce a machine that would think. It was a natural extension, therefore, following World War II for psychologists to use the concepts of information theory to study the brain.[2,3] The proposition was not that the digital computer is a good model of the brain because in many ways it is not. The argument was more subtle and more powerful; a digital computer is an information processing system and the brain is an information processing system, thus the general principles that apply to all information processing systems will apply to both. Study of digital computers and telecommunication reveals the general principles that can then be applied to the brain.

1. Information processing systems have a finite capacity.
2. Information is processed in noise and it is not possible to reduce the error rate to zero.
3. The components of information processing systems are subject to the laws of entropy and will decay in performance with time (age). This means that the error rate will rise with time.
4. Information systems use redundancy to reduce the error rate. Highly complicated information processing systems would have an unexpectedly high error rate in the absence of redundancy.

The brain is obviously an information processing system and these general principles will apply in studying its performance. It is my contention that other biological systems can be regarded as information processing. This certainly applies to the immune system.[4] At birth infants are presented with a vast array of micro-organisms bearing surface epitopes. The immune system has the task of analysing these epitopes, classifying them into self and non-self and then initiating an appropriate response. The system has a finite capacity and this is most likely to be exceeded early in life when many new epitopes are presented. The information is processed in noise and errors will occur even in an otherwise fully functional system. Errors will predispose to infection or to autoimmune disease.

This risk of error will rise with age and it is shown below that these general principles can be used to develop models that explain the age incidence of infectious and autoimmune disease.

The other systems of the body can also be regarded as information processing systems. For instance the control of blood glucose involves the complex interaction of many different genetic systems concerned with food absorption, metabolism and insulin production. Maintaining a constant blood glucose level involves information flow between all these components. Equally the maintenance of blood flow at the appropriate pressure in arteries and veins involves the complex co-ordination of heart muscle action, endothelial integrity and the production of pro and anti-coagulant cytokines. The system could not work without a complex flow of information and components for detecting change and responding appropriately.

AGEING

The general principles of information theory indicate that any system that processes information and makes decisions in an uncertain world is subject to the laws of entropy. Performance in individual systems will deteriorate with time and the error rate will rise. Deterioration and decay in the system is a random process and in biological organisms this is ultimately due to loss of information in the DNA code as a result of somatic mutation. The occurrence of redundancy, however, influences the rate of decay. In a highly redundant system performance falls off slowly initially but then starts to accelerate. It is possible to model this process with a simple mathematical function. Let R be the probability that a single system makes a correct decision. Then $1-R$ is the probability that a single system makes an incorrect decision. Let us assume that R falls exponentially with time i.e. it undergoes random decay. The probability of error at time t is then $1 - Re^{-kt}$ where e is the exponential function and k is a constant governing the rate of decay. Now consider n identical independent systems working in parallel. An error in this system will only occur if all n systems make the same mistake at the same time. The chance of error at time t is now $(1 - Re^{-kt})^n$. With a suitable choice of constants this function closely approximates to the observed relationship between probability of death and age in humans (Fig. 11.1). A plot of risk of dying against age on a log scale gives a straight line with a slope of seven (Fig. 11.2). The slope of the line is a product of redundancy, the higher the degree of redundancy the steeper the slope. The number seven is therefore related to the level of redundancy in the human genome.[5]

The concept of ageing is that all systems are undergoing decay at random and therefore the risk of degenerative disease will increase with age following a similar function to that of death. In fact ischaemic heart disease, degenerative lung disease, the majority of common cancers and infections of old age such as bronchopneumonia all show an exponential increase with age similar to that of the risk of dying. Whichever disease strikes first is a product of chance, lifestyle and genetic constitution. The only way to influence the process and slow down the rate of ageing is to adopt a lifestyle that reduces the constant k in the function $(1 - Re^{-kt})^n$. A challenge for pathology is to find ways of measuring k that are presumably related to the rate of somatic mutation i.e. the rate of decay in the genetic code.

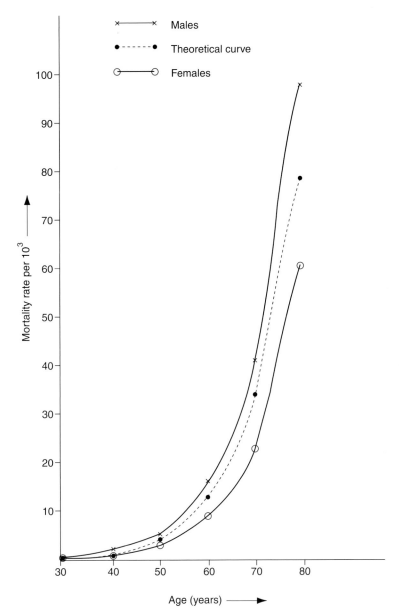

Fig. 11.1 The mortality rate by age for men (x–x) and women (o–o) in England and Wales together with a theoretical curve (•- - - -•) generated by the function $(1 - Re^{-kt})^n$.

AUTOIMMUNITY AND INFECTION

The immune system is presented with a vast array of micro-organisms on mucosal surfaces such as the gastro-intestinal tract and the respiratory tract. Each micro-organism has a range of surface epitopes, some of which are similar to those of host cells (molecular mimicry). This vast range of epitopes is information that must be processed, analysed and responded to in order to protect the host from disease. Errors in information processing will increase the risk of disease.

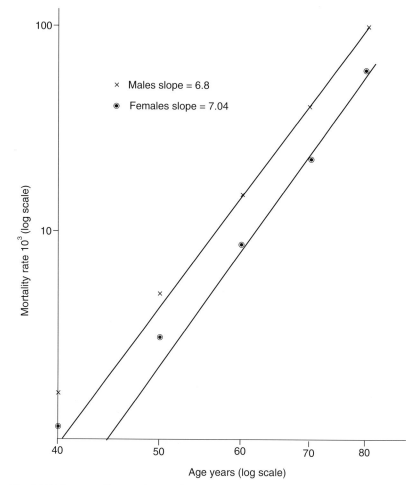

Fig. 11.2 The mortality rate by age for men (x) and women (⊙) in England and Wales plotted on a log scale. The maximum slope is 6.8 for males and 7.04 for females.

Failure to mount an adequate response to a foreign epitope increases the risk of invasive infection by the micro-organism carrying that epitope. Conversely failure to recognize that a particular epitope on a micro-organism is similar to a host epitope increases the risk of autoimmune disease.

The risk of error in information processing rises exponentially with age as shown in the previous section. The age incidence of first exposure to any single common micro-organism falls exponentially with age. For instance if 50% of infants and children meet a particular micro-organism in any one year then 50% will be exposed for the first time in the first year of life, 25% (–50% of the remaining 50%) will be exposed for the first time in the second year of life, 12.5% in the third year and so on. The risk of infection and autoimmune disease that occurs on first exposure is then the resultant of two curves, one falling with time and one rising with time. This is illustrated in Fig. 11.3.

Infectious mononucleosis and paralytic poliomyelitis both illustrate the principle that the age incidence of disease is different from the age incidence of first exposure to the relevant micro-organisms. Infectious mononucleosis is caused by

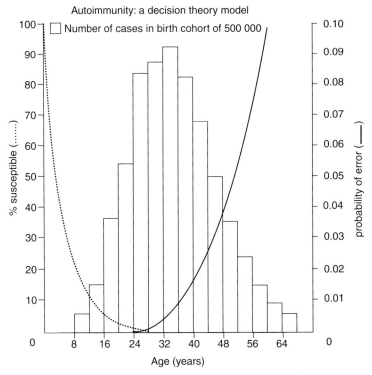

Fig. 11.3 Theoretical age distribution histogram of autoimmune or infectious disease produced by a rising error function interacting with a falling curve of susceptibility.

a common virus that most children meet early in life. Early exposure leads to a mild inapparent infection in most cases i.e. the host makes appropriate decisions and quickly gets control of the infecting organism. Those individuals who are exposed for the first time in the late teenage years are much more likely to suffer a severe symptomatic infection i.e. the increased risk of error in information processing leads to a sub-optimal response and the disease is more severe. Exposure to poliovirus, in the pre-immunization era, showed similar features. Early exposure in infancy usually caused a mild inapparent infection. Later exposure led to an increased risk of severe disease and paralysis.

A number of autoimmune diseases show an age incidence curve that rises to a peak in the middle years and then falls. Examples include multiple sclerosis (Fig. 11.4), psoriasis, thyrotoxicosis, insulin dependent diabetes mellitus (IDDM) and rheumatic fever. In the case of multiple sclerosis the peak is in the third decade, in psoriasis it is late in the second decade and in IDDM it is early in the second decade. It is possible to produce models of the age incidence of each of these conditions using the information model (see Fig. 11.4 for multiple sclerosis). The basic assumption is that the conditions are precipitated by first exposure to a micro-organism bearing a specific epitope that shows molecular mimicry to host tissue. There is good evidence for this idea in the case of rheumatic fever and varying degrees of supporting evidence in the other conditions. The principle of modelling disease incidence is shown in Fig. 11.3. A falling curve, determined by first exposure to a micro-organism, interacts with a rising curve, determined by the ageing process, to produce the disease curve which rises to a peak in the

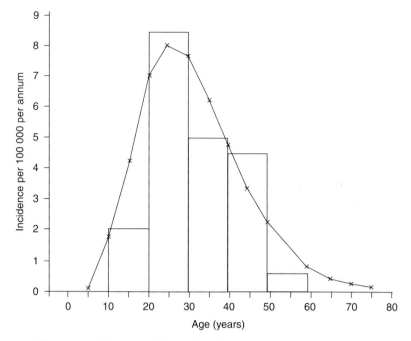

Fig. 11.4 A histogram of the age incidence of multiple sclerosis together with a theoretical curve (x–x) produced by the information theory model.

middle years. If the micro-organism is common the first curve falls rapidly and the disease peaks early. If the organism is less common the first curve falls more slowly and the disease peaks later. Thus for multiple sclerosis, knowing the age incidence of the disease and knowing the rate of ageing, the model predicts that the micro-organism is one that 25% of the population encounter in any one year.[6] The organisms causing IDDM and rheumatic fever are much more common. In the case of IDDM the disease does not present clinically until most of the B cells in the pancreas have been destroyed. The first wave of attack on the B cells obviously occurs much earlier, perhaps in the first few years of life, in which case the initiating micro-organisms must be very common indeed.[7]

STATISTICAL DECISION THEORY

The process of making decisions in an uncertain world is the subject of statistical decision theory.[8]

Consider the problem of a man viewing a radar screen and trying to decide whether or not a signal has occurred. Figure 11.5 plots frequency and intensity for signal and noise in this situation. Even in the absence of a signal photons will emerge from any point on the screen and the number of photons emerging is a random variable. The frequency distribution of photons in the absence of a signal constitutes background noise. If a signal occurs many more photons emerge, but once again the number is a random variable. The decision problem is to set a threshold level of intensity such that all values above it are judged to be a signal and all values below it are judged to be noise. Since signal and noise are random

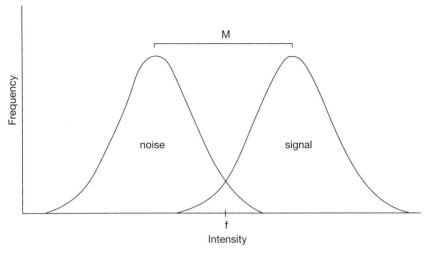

Fig. 11.5 Frequency distribution of signal and noise: The signal is of intensity *M* and is superimposed on background noise. If signal and noise are equally likely a decision threshold placed at f will minimize but not eliminate errors.

variables their frequency distributions overlap and wherever the threshold is set errors will occur. The problem for statistical decision theory is to define the factors that influence where the threshold should be set.

One approach is to place the threshold at *f* (Fig. 11.5). This seems intuitively reasonable as it seems to minimize the number of incorrect responses. This is true only if signal and noise are equally likely. If noise is much more likely than signal the threshold needs to be moved to the right in order to minimize incorrect responses. Thus if the goal of the decision strategy is to be right most of the time one must consider the evidence (the number of photons) and the *a priori* probability (the relative likelihood of signal and noise prior to observation).

Table 11.2 shows that there are four types of response.

1. A correct positive i.e. respond signal given that a signal occurred.
2. A correct negative i.e. respond noise given no signal.
3. A false positive i.e. respond signal given noise.
4. A false negative i.e. respond noise given signal.

Table 11.2 shows *w* correct positives, *z* correct negatives, *y* false positives and *x* false negatives. The following definitions are worth committing to memory as they are becoming increasingly important in a number of areas of histopathological practice such as audit of breast fine needle aspirates and cervical cytology.

Table 11.2 The table shows *w* correct positives, *z* correct negatives, *x* false negatives, and *y* false positives in a detection system that attempts to distinguish signal (S) from noise (N).

| | Response | | |
	S	N	Totals
True/S	w	x	w+x
True/N	y	z	y+z
Totals	w+y	x+z	w+x+y+z

- Sensitivity = the probability of a correct positive response = $\dfrac{w}{w+x}$
- Specificity = the probability of a correct negative response = $\dfrac{z}{y+z}$
- Predictive value of a positive response = the probability that a positive response is correct = $\dfrac{w}{w+y}$
- Predictive value of a negative response = the probability that a negative response is correct = $\dfrac{z}{x+z}$

In the radar problem if the threshold is moved to the right the probability of a false positive is reduced but the probability of a false negative increases. If the threshold is moved to the left false positives become more common and false negatives less common. It is a general principle of decision theory that attempts to reduce one type of error will inevitably increase the opposite type of error. A plot of the probability of a correct positive (sensitivity) against the probability of a false positive (1 – specificity) produces a receiver operating curve (ROC) (Fig. 11.6). Moving the threshold so as to increase the probability of a true positive automatically increases the probability of a false positive.

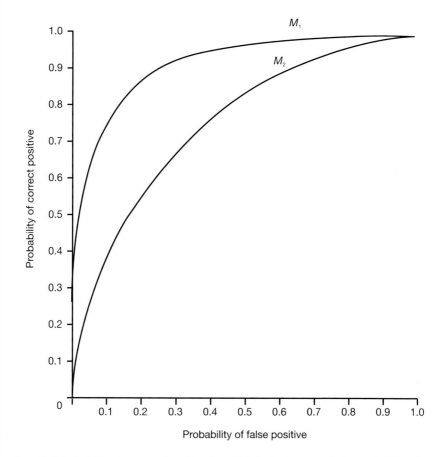

Fig. 11.6 Probability of a correct positive (sensitivity) plotted against the probability of a false positive (1 – specificity) for two values of M where $M_1 > M_2$.

If the goal of a decision strategy is to reduce the number of errors then the *a priori* probability and evidence need to be taken into consideration in determining the threshold position. In making decisions, however, it is also necessary to consider the consequences of actions that follow from the decision. This is certainly true in biology where decision leads to response. In the radar problem a false negative i.e. failure to recognize a signal, could have disastrous consequences. Failure to recognize and respond to an enemy attack could mean that lives are lost. This is obviously an error to avoid. A false positive, by comparison, is more of an inconvenience. It would lead to an increased state of readiness for attack and preparations that are unnecessary. The penalty of a false negative is obviously greater than a false positive and the threshold needs to be moved to the left. An optimum decision, one that maximizes expected value takes into account (i) *a priori* probability, (ii) evidence, (iii) utility (the values and cost associated with correct and incorrect decisions).

A hypothetical game illustrates the problem of integrating the *a priori* probability, the evidence and the utility into a single decision. You are placed in the centre of a room with the exit behind you. In front of you is a screen and behind it is a short corridor leading to two doors. Behind one door is a man-eating lion, behind the other is a man with a cheque made out to you for £1 000 000. A die is thrown and if the number six appears the lion is released, if any other number appears the man with the cheque is released. You do not know the result of the die cast and have a few seconds to judge from sound and smell whether the lion or the man is approaching. You cannot see behind the screen and if you wait until you can see the lion there will be no time to escape. If you leave and the man is free you forfeit the £1 000 000. The decision involves:

1. The *a priori* probability – in this case it is five times more likely that the man is free than the lion is free.
2. The evidence – this is limited to sound and smell.
3. The utility – this is your subjective judgement of the relative worth of your life and £1 000 000.

The decision will be influenced strongly by utility. For most people, particularly those happily married with a good job and a reasonable income, £1 000 000 will not add a great deal to their total happiness. The best decision is to get out quickly. But if you are a tramp, homeless and depressed with no money and were contemplating suicide anyway, £1 000 000 could transform your life. In which case it is sensible to stay and take a chance. Thus the best decision, the one that maximizes expected value is subjective and will vary from individual to individual.

The various elements of decision theory can be combined into a single decision rule. Consider two hypotheses h_0 and h_1, in the radar problem h_1 might be the hypothesis that a signal occurred, while h_0 is the hypothesis that no signal occurred. The response that maximizes expected value is:

$$L_{10}(e) > B,$$

$$\text{where } L_{10}(e) = \frac{P[e/h_1]}{P[e/h_0]}$$

$$B = \frac{V_{00} + V_{01}}{V_{11} + V_{10}} \frac{P[h_0]}{P[h_1]}$$

$L_{10}(e)$ is the likelihood ratio of event e for h_1 relative to h_0.

$P[e/h_1]$ is the probability of event e given h_1.

$P[e/h_0]$ is the probability of event e given h_0.

$P[h_0]$ is the *a priori* probability of h_0.

$P[h_1]$ is the *a priori* probability of h_1.

V_{00} is the value of choosing h_0 given h_0.

V_{01} is the cost of choosing h_1 given h_0.

V_{11} is the value of choosing h_1 given h_1.

V_{10} is the cost of choosing h_0 given h_1.

This notation may appear confusing but the idea is relatively simple. In the radar problem the intensity of light is measured (event e) and the likelihood ratio is calculated as the probability of event e given h_1 divided by the probability of event e given h_0. The threshold is set at B, which is determined by the *a priori* probability of h_1 and h_0 and the values and costs associated with correct and incorrect responses. If $L_{10}(e)$ exceeds B hypothesis h_1 is accepted over h_0.

Concepts from statistical decision theory are directly relevant to day-to-day practice in histopathology.

1. Histopathologists need to know how to define sensitivity, specificity and the predictive values and use them in audit of cervical cytology and breast fine needle aspirates.
2. We must realize that altering criteria in order to reduce false positive diagnoses will automatically increase false negatives and vice versa.
3. The decisions we make are not just based on morphological appearance but also should take into account the *a priori* probability. All histopathologists have had the experience of making a diagnosis on morphology alone and subsequently learning of clinical details that make another diagnosis more likely. In our practice clinical information sets the *a priori* probability for our decisions. Diagnoses made without that information will be sub-optimal. This principle needs to be borne in mind when histological diagnoses are reviewed. The morphological evidence is the same on review but the *a priori* probability will have changed.
4. The optimum decision strategy is not to seek to minimize error but to maximize expected value. In cervical cytology false positives create anxiety and lead to unnecessary surgical procedures but false negatives can mean failure to prevent invasive cancer. The optimum strategy is not to obtain the least number of mistakes but to do the least harm to, or most good for, the patient.

MORPHOLOGICAL CLASSIFICATION

Histopathologists classify disease using morphological patterns. There are two types of classification that need to be distinguished. Nominal classification involves the recognition of different entities. For instance breast carcinoma and fibroadenoma need to be clearly distinguished and most histopathologists will go through a professional career without confusing one for the other. Using systems of nominal classification it is possible to recognize hundreds, if not thousands, of different entities. If the classification criteria are clear and objective the diagnoses are reliable and most histopathologists would agree on the diagnosis in any specific case. Biological variability means that a degree of overlap can occur between what are otherwise well defined discrete entities and there will be a degree of uncertainty in a few problem cases. Overall, however, the systems of nominal classification work well. Ordinal classification involves classification along a continuum. For instance colonic carcinoma can be well or moderately or poorly differentiated. This is a continuum of change and the divisions between grades are arbitrary. In this situation disagreement between observers will occur. A practical question is how many grades should be used?

One approach to this problem has been to use kappa statistics, which measure the degree of agreement between observers having corrected for chance.

$$\kappa = \frac{P(A) - P(E)}{1 - P(E)}$$

κ = Kappa coefficient of agreement.

P(A) = the proportion of times the observers agree.

P(E) = the proportion of times the observers would agree purely by chance.

In general if the number of categories is decreased the degree of inter-observer agreement increases and this has been used as an argument for fewer categories. For instance if three categories of dyskaryosis are used in the assessment of cervical smears (mild, moderate and severe) there is less agreement than if two categories (low and high grade) are used. The problem is, of course, that if only one category were used there would be even more agreement but the information transmitted to the surgeon would be less.[9]

Another approach is to measure the amount of information transmitted. Consider a dot placed at random between two markers (Fig. 11.7). The pathologist observes the figure and tells the clinician where the dot is placed. If the pathologist uses two categories i.e. first and second half and tells the clinician accurately which half it is in then one bit of information is transmitted. Initially there are two possibilities, after the information is received there is one possibility and the uncertainty has been reduced by a half. If the pathologist uses four categories (first quarter, second quarter, third quarter and fourth quarter) and tells the clinician accurately which quarter it is in then two bits of information are transmitted (uncertainty reduced from 4 to 1 and $\log_2 4 = 2$). If eight categories are used and the position is noted accurately then three bits of information are transmitted.

The problem is that as more categories are used the pathologist is more likely to misclassify the position and the amount of information transmitted is less than the maximum that could be transmitted. Experiments of this type have been performed many times, not using pathologists and clinicians, but asking subjects to estimate along a single dimension.[3] The amount of information transmitted increases as the number of response categories is increased up to a maximum of approximately seven. Thereafter increasing the number of categories does not increase information transmission but importantly neither does it decrease it. These experiments indicate that at least seven categories should be used for maximum information transmission.

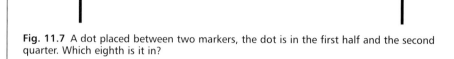

Fig. 11.7 A dot placed between two markers, the dot is in the first half and the second quarter. Which eighth is it in?

The use of seven categories fits naturally into most of our grading systems. For instance cervical smears are normally classified on a four point scale as normal, mild dyskaryosis, moderate dyskaryosis or severe dyskaryosis. Everyone who reports smears knows, however, that the difficulty is not recognizing the classical four but dealing with the ones in between. We recognize borderline between normal and mild dyskaryosis, but also degrees of dyskaryosis somewhere between mild and moderate or moderate and severe. In practice we use a seven point scale (four main categories and three in between). A similar situation occurs in grading tumours. There are four main types i.e. well differentiated, moderately differentiated, poorly differentiated and undifferentiated. In addition there are the ones between giving seven in all.

The electromagnetic spectrum is a continuum but we recognize seven colours in the rainbow. This is not a property of the spectrum but a property of the way in which our brains analyse the spectrum. Equally there are seven tones on a musical scale (seven steps in an octave). Miller wrote a classical paper entitled 'the magical number seven, plus or minus two', in which he pointed out that the number seven keeps reappearing whenever human information processing is measured.[3] Seven items can be held in short term memory, seven categories recognized on a uni-dimensional continuum, and $\log_2 7$ is the amount of information processed when a number of different skills are assessed. Miller wondered whether this was coincidence or the consequence of a deeper design. It is of considerable interest, in this context, that when ageing is analysed in terms of information the number seven reappears as the level of redundancy in information processing (Fig. 11.2).

Seven categories applies to a uni-dimensional continuum. In theory it is possible to increase information transmission above $\log_2 7$ bits if more than one dimension is used. For instance breast tumours could be assessed for pleomorphism (seven point scale), mitotic activity (seven point scale) and tubule formation (seven point scale). Integrating these assessments could increase the number of categories beyond seven. Visual assessment of coronary artery stenosis commonly uses a percentage scale (100 response categories), but in practice only seven will be reliably distinguished. If a series of standard photographs of 10%, 20%, 30%, 40%, 50%, 60%, 70%, 80% and 90% stenosis are available the visual assessment could in theory be seven categories within the 10% limits. If a number of individuals independently assess a uni-dimensional continuum this is equivalent to assessing an entity on a number of different dimensions. Thus the mean assessment of several individuals will lead to more than seven categories being reliably judged. Thus it is possible, in theory, to increase the precision of subjective judgements in histopathology by (i) using more than one dimension of assessment, (ii) using visual standards, (iii) averaging the results of several independent observers. Little experimental work has been carried out in histopathology on ways of improving the precision of subjective judgements using information theory and this is a fertile area for a numerate trainee in histopathology to explore.

REDUNDANCY AND SEX

Redundancy is a very important property of information processing systems. When information is analysed it is important that there are checks and double checks in order to reduce the risk of error to a minimum. By taking in more information than the maximum required and by checking and re-checking the analysis the effect mathematically is equivalent to reducing the variance of the signal and noise frequency distributions in Fig. 11.5. This reduces overlap and thereby reduces the frequency of false positives and false negatives. Redundancy does not eliminate error but it reduces it. All information processing systems contain components that are at risk of error and breakdown. As complexity increases and the number of components increases the risk of error will rise. Thus as systems become more complicated higher and higher levels of redundancy are required.

Biological organisms are coded by genes. If a single gene codes for a single component of a highly redundant complex system the effect of a deleterious mutation involving the gene will have a negligible effect on performance. Thus there cannot be strong selective pressure acting against single mutations in a complex genetic system. The only way that selection can act is against combinations of deleterious mutations which interact synergistically to impair performance.

An interesting property of redundancy is that loss of several components in a redundant system can lead to synergistic interaction.[10] Consider the example of a secretary checking through a letter to correct typographical errors. Let us assume that there is a 0.1 chance of a particular error being undetected. If seven secretaries check the letter, all acting independently, a highly redundant system, the chance that the error is undetected is $(0.1)^7 = 10^{-7}$. If one secretary is lost and there are six checks the chance the error is undetected is 10^{-6}, this is a tenfold rise but in absolute terms the difference is negligible. If five checks are made the chance of error is 10^{-5} and so on. This is shown in Fig. 11.8. The effect of losing one or two components in a redundant system is negligible, but then in one or two more steps the error rate can become significant.

The theoretical argument for redundancy in the genome is compelling, but there is also now some empirical evidence in support of this idea. When the genome of brewer's yeast (*Saccharomyces cerevisiae*) was sequenced many were surprised to discover a high degree of redundancy.[11] More recently there is evidence that up to four new mutations have entered the human genome in each generation since humans and chimpanzees evolved from a common ancestor six million years ago.[12] The human race could not have survived without some system for selecting against combinations of deleterious mutations.

The model that has been used to analyse this problem is as follows. Assume there are N independent complex highly redundant information processing systems in the human genome. The mean number of deleterious mutations in the

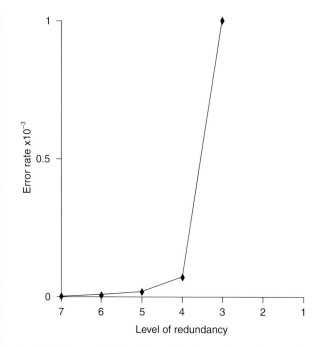

Fig. 11.8 The probability of error in a letter rises as the number of proof readers is reduced.

zygote of individuals who survive to contribute to the next generation is Y. The mean number of new deleterious mutations that arise in each generation and are passed to the next generation is X. The deleterious mutations are distributed at random in N systems. One or two deleterious mutations per system has no effect on function. If there are several mutations in a system then the function is severely impaired and there will be selection against that individual at the zygote stage or later leading to genetic death (failure to pass on genes to the next generation). If there is an intermediate number of deleterious mutations in a system then the system is impaired but not fatally, that individual is likely to survive but suffer polygenic impairment of function. It is possible that this will not become manifest till later in life when other systems deteriorate.

The precursor cells of spermatozoa and oocytes have an average of $Y+X$ deleterious mutations. In meiosis the mutations are distributed at random to gametes and then the gametes fuse at random during sexual reproduction to form zygotes. Thus in the next generation of zygotes the number of deleterious mutations in zygotes will show a Poisson distribution (approximately) with a mean of $Y+X$. The zygotes at the upper end of the Poisson distribution are more likely to have systems with several mutations and are therefore less likely to survive. Thus a subset of zygotes survive to contribute to the next generation and the mean number of mutations in the sub-set is Y. The models that have been developed indicate that 25% to 75% of zygotes that form will survive and there is some empirical data which supports this. Couples engaging in regular unprotected sexual intercourse have a 25% chance of producing a viable zygote in any one menstrual cycle.

This model is still under active development and not all implications have been fully explored. One interesting aspect is that the model explains why sexual reproduction is so much more successful than asexual reproduction. In an organism that is exclusively asexual new deleterious mutations will accumulate in the genome through successive generations leading to eventual extinction. A sexual phase, however, distributes the deleterious mutations unevenly in the next generation and a few organisms with low levels of mutations can survive. This means that survival in sexually reproducing organisms depends on generating and exploiting inequality.

An area of concern for health professionals is the uneven distribution of health and disease in society. Certain sections of the population bear a disproportionate share of ill-health and premature death. The diseases involved include common conditions such as ischaemic heart disease, which are traditionally viewed as having a polygenic component. It could be that part of the health inequality is due to the random process by which deleterious mutations are distributed during sexual reproduction. Those individuals who are lucky enough to receive a small number are more likely to do well in all aspects of biological endeavour including fighting disease and maintaining the integrity of their systems into old age.

The value of X will presumably vary in different cultures and at different times. If social conditions improve with better diets presumably mutation rates could fall. Conversely increased industrial pollution and exposure to chemical carcinogens and radiation could cause the mutation rate to rise. In societies where X is low the value of Y will fall and the entire population will be healthier with increased longevity. If X rises the health of future generations will suffer. Methods for measuring and monitoring mutation rates in the general population are required in order to identify those lifestyles that lead to the lowest rates of mutation.

CONCLUSION

The concept of information is of both practical and theoretical interest in pathology. Statistical decision theory has established the principles that underlie the process of making decisions in an uncertain world. It is impossible to completely avoid error and histopathologists need to be aware of the relationship between false positives and false negatives. Definitions of sensitivity, specificity and positive and negative predictive values are increasingly being used in audit. The goal of a decision strategy should not be to reduce errors to a minimum but to maximize expected value. This involves considering (i) the *a priori* probability, (ii) the evidence and (iii) the utility, in all diagnoses. Evidence alone is not enough and making morphological diagnoses in the absence of clinical information and in ignorance of management options will lead to bad decisions. When histopathological slides are reviewed it is important to remember that the morphological appearance is only part of the diagnosis, not the whole of it.

An important practical question in histopathology is how many grades can be recognized along a continuum of change? The amount of information transmitted rises to a maximum with seven categories but the degree of observer agreement falls as the number of categories is increased. In theory the amount of information transmitted could be increased by (i) analysing the morphological appearance along more than one dimension, (ii) combining the judgements of several independent observers, (iii) using photographic standards to define points along the continuum. This is an area in which more research is needed.

A possible explanation of the age incidence of autoimmune disease in terms of interaction between first exposure to common micro-organisms and a rising error curve is an extremely useful product of information theory. In the case of IDDM the micro-organisms must be very common and this implicates bacteria of the normal microbial flora. If the micro-organisms that precipitate autoimmune disease could be identified it would be an important step on the way to prevention.

The steady loss of information from the genetic code due to the accumulation of deleterious mutations would lead to extinction of the species if there were not some method, such as sexual reproduction, to divide the deleterious mutations unequally between the progeny. Individuals with the least number of deleterious mutations survive to maintain the species. A similar process of steady loss of information from the genetic code occurs in individuals due to somatic mutation. In this case the process cannot be reversed and leads to ageing and death. A challenge for pathology is to develop simple inexpensive methods for measuring mutation rates in cells and apply them to monitor the general population. Defining lifestyles that reduce mutation rates would slow down the process of ageing and increase the health of future generations.

KEY POINT

1. Information is a fundamental concept, which like energy in physics, could play an important role in defining the theoretical basis of biology. The general principles that apply to all systems that process information will apply to many of the complex areas of biological behaviour.
2. Modelling the process of decay in a highly complex highly redundant system leads to a relationship between error and time that matches that between death and age in humans. The interaction between this error curve and the age at first exposure to micro-organisms can then explain age incidence curves seen in autoimmune disease.
3. Redundancy in the human genome combined with a new deleterious mutation rate exceeding one per generation means that selection must act against the combination of deleterious mutations that show synergistic interaction. This model, which is still under active development, has implications for concepts of polygenic disease, the relationship between polygenic disease and environmental mutagenesis, and health inequality.
4. Statistical decision theory is concerned with the process of making optimum decisions in an uncertain world. It defines the relationship between true and false positives and true and false negatives and this is increasingly important in histopathological audit. An optimum decision depends on (i) the *a priori* probability, (ii) the evidence, and (iii) the values and costs associated with correct and incorrect decisions (utility). All these factors need to be taken into account when framing histopathological diagnoses.
5. The amount of information transmitted by the pathologist to the clinician can be estimated using information theory. A large amount of information can be transmitted using systems of nominal classification if the entities are clearly defined. In systems of ordinal classification along a continuum the amount of information transmitted is limited (approximately $\log_2 7$ bits) and a degree of

inter-observer disagreement is inevitable. In theory, however, information transmission could be increased by (i) analysing along more than one dimension, (ii) combining the judgements of several observers, (iii) using photographic standards that define points on the continuum.

REFERENCES

1. Shannon CE. The mathematical theory of communication. Bell Syst Technol J 1948; 27: 379–423
2. Cherry C. On Human Communication. Cambridge, Massachusetts MIT Press: 1957
3. Miller GA. The Psychology of Communication. London: Penguin Press 1968
4. Morris J A. Autoimmunity: a decision theory model. J Clin Pathol 1987; 40: 210–215
5. Morris JA. Ageing, information and the magical number seven. Med Hypoth 1992; 39: 291–294
6. Morris JA. The age incidence of multiple sclerosis: a decision theory model. Med Hypoth 1990; 32: 129–135
7. Morris JA. A possible role for bacteria in the pathogenesis of insulin dependent diabetes mellitus. Med Hypoth 1989; 29: 231–235
8. Green DM, Swets JA. Signal detection theory and psychophysics. London: John Wiley and Sons, 1966
9. Morris JA. Information and observer disagreement in histopathology. Histopathology 1994; 25: 123–128
10. Morris JA. Genetic control of redundant systems. Med Hypoth 1997; 49: 159–164
11. Oliver SG. From DNA sequence to biological function. Nature 1996; 379: 597–600
12. Eyre-Walker A, Keightley P D. High genomic mutation rates in hominoids. Nature 1999; 397: 344–347

Index

Indexer: Dr Laurence Errington

B

B–cell chronic lymphocytic
leukaemia *see* lymphocytic
leukaemia
B–cell lymphomas, cutaneous 1–16
B–lymphoblastic lymphoma 12
Barrett, Norman 59
Barrett's oesophagus (and
columnar lined
oesophagus; CLO) 57–80
cytology 72
dysplasia in 66–67
epidemiology 58
histology 62–63, 67–68
treatment effects 73–74
historical perspectives and
definitions 59–60
metaplasia–dysplasia–cancer
sequence *see*
adenocarcinoma;
dysplasia; metaplasia
molecular pathology 68–72
pathogenesis/aetiology 61–62
short segment/ultra–short
segment CLO (SSCLO;
USSCLO) 60, 62, 64–65
surveillance controversy 75–76
basement membrane disorders,
skin 103, 112–116
bile reflux 61
biopsies, gastric, non–neoplastic,
routine reporting 121–134
blistering disorders 110–111,
112–116
blood flow, arterial
decreased 139–140, 144, 146–147
increased 139, 144
blood pressure, high *see*
hypertension
blood vessel structure 135–152
normal 135–139
pathology (structural
alterations/remodelling)
138–149
diagnostic pointers and pitfalls
145–148
Bragg reflection 83–84
brush cytology, Barrett's
oesophagus 72

bullous (blistering) disorders
110–111, 112–116
bullous pemphigoid antigen–2
115

C

cadherin and Barrett's oesophagus
70–71
calcium ion pump gene, mutation
111–112
cancer *see* malignant tumours
carcinoma, oesophageal (in
Barrett's oesophagus) *see*
adenocarcinoma
catenin and Barrett's oesophagus
71
CD antigens (cutaneous
lymphoproliferative
disease diagnosis) 2
B–cell chronic lymphocytic
leukaemia 13
B–lymphoblastic lymphoma 12
follicle centre lymphoma 4
immunocytoma 8
intravascular large B–cell
lymphoma 12
marginal zone lymphoma 6
plasmacytoma 10
CD44 and Barrett's oesophagus 71
cell
adhesion *see* adhesion
arteries
growth *see* growth
injury responses 142–143
cephalic histiocytosis, benign 37
chemical gastritis 130
children
histiocytosis
Langherhans' cell 31, 32
non–Langherhans' cell 34, 37
spring eruption 20
chronic lymphocytic leukaemia *see*
lymphocytic leukaemia
CMV gastritis 132
collagen type VII mutation in
dystrophic epidermolysis
bullosa 114
computed tomography, micro